Evaluation of Therapeutic Recreation Through Quality Assurance

ATRA

EVALUATION OF THERAPEUTIC RECREATION THROUGH QUALITY ASSURANCE

Edited by

BOB RILEY

Assistant Professor
Department of Recreation and Leisure Studies
Green Mountain College
Poultney, Vermont

VENTURE PUBLISHING, INC.

State College, PA

Cover Design by Sandra Sikorski
Design and Copy Editing by Susan Lewis
Production Supervision by Bonnie Godbey
Library of Congress Catalogue Card Number 87-50299
ISBN 0-910251-18-5

NOTES FROM THE ATRA PUBLICATION COMMITTEE

The Publication Committee of the American Therapeutic Recreation Association is pleased to make available to practicing professionals their *Evaluation of Therapeutic Recreation through Quality Assurance.* This publication represents a milestone for the American Therapeutic Recreation Association and the therapeutic recreation profession in general.

For the American Therapeutic Recreation Association, this is the first official publication that they have offered to the profession. In turn, *Evaluation of Therapeutic Recreation through Quality Assurance* enables them to serve the profession by yet another means.

For professionals, *Evaluation of Therapeutic Recreation through Quality Assurance* offers state-of-the-art information of a theoretical and practical nature. At a time when accountability is of paramount importance to quality health care, our professional organizations must offer practitioners the most current data and techniques. *Evaluation of Therapeutic Recreation through Quality Assurance* meets this objective.

Thomas K. Skalko
Publication Chair
University of Southern Mississippi

TABLE OF CONTENTS

FOREWORD

PREFACE

ACKNOWLEDGEMENTS

CONTRIBUTORS

FOREWORD

It was with a great deal of pleasure that I participated in "Evaluation of Therapeutic Recreation through Quality Assurance." As a music therapist who is employed as a program manager within the Department of Education Programs at the Joint Commission on Accreditation of Hospitals (JCAH), my job primarily involves managing and teaching quality-assurance-related seminars. The therapeutic recreation profession's proactive stance to this extremely important and timely topic is most impressive. During the three days of the conference it was clear that both the presenters and the participants were successful in identifying the role that quality assurance currently plays in the provision of therapeutic recreation, and in developing a strategy for building upon that foundation. These proceedings should be extremely helpful to all members of the therapeutic recreation profession as an excellent overview of relevant quality-assurance issues.

The presenters emphasized that in today's health environment we are now witnessing the pendulum swinging back from concerns of cost accountability to concerns of quality accountability. Quality assurance is the mechanism by which the therapeutic recreation professional can be accountable for quality and appropriate service. Accountability will enable therapeutic recreation professionals to establish the need for their services, demonstrate the quality and appropriateness of care, determine the therapeutic effect of service, and validate the resources necessary for excellent care.

Defining quality will require clearly delineated organizational structures, management processes, and clinical outcome components. If therapeutic recreation professionals cannot define what constitutes quality in the services they offer, then other health-care groups will probably do it for them. (These could include the government, business, third-party payers, and/or consumers.) Possibly, if therapeutic recreation services are not adequately defined, then health-care consumers could also choose other activity-related services that *have* quality-defined services and are therefore viewed as more accountable.

Quality assurance is also a very timely topic for the JCAH. The Joint Committee has recently adopted an agenda for change in an attempt to launch a new perspective for quality assurance in health care. The central purpose of this agenda is to assure that patients and the quality of their care remain the principal concern of a health-care delivery system that is characterized by economic competition, resource limitations, and new and unmonitored delivery systems. The centerpiece of this agenda calls for the development of severely adjusted measurements of clinical outcomes and the incorporation of these measurements into a new and more relevant survey process. This endeavor will require the assistance of the entire health-care field, including therapeutic recreation.

In view of the above developments, this conference has been successful in providing therapeutic recreation professionals with the opportunity to identify and share information regarding state-of-the-art quality-assurance efforts. These conference proceedings should prove beneficial to all therapeutic recreation professionals, educators, and students who are concerned with being accountable to their peers, other health care professionals, and, most importantly, to their patients.

To my knowledge, this endeavor is far beyond anything that other activity-related professionals have accomplished. Admittedly, defining quality within a professional context is a very difficult and consuming task. The therapeutic recreation profession, as all other health-care professions, will need to devote much time, energy, and resources to achieve a recognized level of accountability. These proceedings will provide an excellent framework for achieving this goal.

Richard W. Scalenghe, RMT
Program Manager
Department of Education Programs
Joint Commission on Accreditation of Hospitals

PREFACE

Quality assurance (QA) is one of the most pervasive topics in the health-care industry today. In light of the emphasis placed upon prospective pricing and revised regulatory standards, concern for the provision of quality care and services is paramount among health-care professionals. This increased emphasis upon the provision of quality health-care stems, to a large degree, from the various elements that constitute the reimbursement component of the health-care industry—third-party payers. In essence, QA has emerged as a prominent issue primarily due to increased efforts to provide more efficient, effective, and cost-contained services.

This book is an effort to address these concerns within the realm of the therapeutic-recreation process. It is the direct outgrowth of the 1986 conference on the "Evaluation of Therapeutic Recreation through Quality Assurance," held at Green Mountain College, Poultney, Vermont. Viewed as a timely and critically informative workshop, the conference explored the need for implementing effective QA programs within therapeutic recreation delivery systems. This book, which is representative of all of the papers presented at the conference, provides a comprehensive look at the therapeutic-recreation QA process from concept through implementation.

While there is general agreement among therapeutic recreation professionals that quality services should be provided, there exists little consensus as to what constitutes quality care and, furthermore, how we should monitor it. Historically, the focus of the accreditation process has been on the structure and process measurements of health-care delivery. JCAH is now convinced that it is both appropriate and necessary to begin looking at the measurement of health-care outcomes. Utilizing only structure and process standards during a survey, the Joint Commission has only been able to determine if a facility did in fact provide quality services. Adopting outcome measures will assure that such services did in fact lead to improved health-care status. Initial efforts to incorporate clinical outcome measurements into the accreditation survey will begin in 1987.

The articles contained within this volume provide a framework by which therapeutic recreation professionals involved in QA can develop their own perspective and strategies in reference to their specific settings. This is not to suggest that QA efforts and strategies within the therapeutic recreation profession should not be consistent. Quite the contrary is true. However, the QA process must be viewed as a two-way exchange between professional standards established on a national basis and individual protocol utilized at a practitioner level. The format and sequence of articles contained within this book reflect this premise.

The first two articles present an overview of the therapeutic-recreation/quality-assurance relationship. In the opening paper, Ray West, President of the American Therapeutic Recreation Association, provides a stimulating argument on the need for quality assurance in therapeutic recreation. Following this introduction, Bob Riley, in the second article, presents a conceptual discussion of quality assurance within the framework of both the professional organization and the practitioner.

Building upon the concepts presented by the first two authors, George Donovan and James Ticehurst, in separate works, discuss QA regulatory issues from a national perspective. In the first of these two papers, Donovan identifies the major regulatory agencies that influence, via standards, the provision of quality services in therapeutic recreation. Ticehurst, as an administrator for the Vermont Professional Review Organization (PRO), provides a firsthand account of the regulatory process of peer review. Additionally, the author provides a stimulating challenge to therapeutic recreation to become involved in the PRO process both from the perspective of ethical concern and professional survival.

In an effort to address the QA process on a more pragmatic basis, the next three authors provide practical guidelines to implement quality-assurance activities. Nancy Navar, from a strategic point of view, presents an informative article on developing a departmental "plan of operation," an essential component of the quality-assurance process. Following suit, Steven Wright, in an illustrative effort, provides a discussion of the various mechanisms of the QA process, including establishing elements of care and designing a data-collection system. In the last of the papers presented, Ann Huston provides an overview of a comprehensive therapeutic recreation quality-assurance program. This QA program was designed by the author and is currently utilized by the Veterans Administration. The concluding section of the book provides a summary review and critique of the conference by Ray West.

Collectively, *Evaluation of Therapeutic Recreation through Quality Assurance* combines theory with application to provide a basic introduction to quality assurance for therapeutic recreators. It is presented humbly, as a beginning. The current emphasis on quality assurance may be a final attempt by regulatory agencies to allow professional organizations, (therapeutic recreation) to justify and regulate themselves. It is this editor's hope that this volume will contribute to such efforts and that the therapeutic recreation profession will be strengthened due, in part, to the efforts of those who contributed to this volume.

The first snowfall, Fall 1986.

Bob Riley
Middletown Springs, Vermont

ACKNOWLEDGEMENTS

The completion of this volume required the assistance, dedication and sincere effort of many individuals. The editor wishes to acknowledge the support of the Life Long Learning Program at Green Mountain College, particularly Douglas Durkee, Director, and James Pollock, Founder. This project would not have been completed without the sponsorship of the New England Therapeutic Recreation Consortium (NETRC), which provided financial support for the original QA conference. Additionally, I wish to recognize several individuals—Peg Connolly, Ray West, Rich Hoffman and Steve Wright—who unselfishly shared both professional and personal insights in an effort to make this book a reality.

Deep appreciation is expressed to the American Therapeutic Recreation Association (ATRA) Board of Directors, along with the Publications Committee, Tom Skalko, Chair. Without the support and confidence of these colleagues, this volume would still be a dream. Additionally, each of the contributors to this volume have the editor's sincere appreciation and respect. The professional commitment and personal sacrifice that each of you experienced did not go unnoticed.

Lastly, to Maria and Devin . . . thank you for understanding.

B.R.

CONTRIBUTORS

GEORGE DONOVAN, M.S., CTRS

Chief, Recreation Services
Veterans Administration Medical
    Center
Northampton, MA

ANN D. HUSTON, CTRS

Chief, Recreation Services
Veterans Administration Medical
    Center
Palo Alto, CA

NANCY NAVAR, Re.D., CTRS

Associate Professor
Department of Recreation and
    Parks
University of Wisconsin-LaCrosse
LaCrosse, WI

BOB RILEY, M.S., CTRS

Assistant Professor
Department of Recreation and
    Leisure Studies
Green Mountain College
Poultney, VT

JAMES J. TICEHURST

Contracts Administrator
Vermont Professional Standards
    Review Organization
South Burlington, VT

RAY WEST, M.S., CTRS

Director of Recreation Therapy
North Carolina Memorial Hospital
Chapel Hill, NC

STEVE WRIGHT, M.S., M.P.A.

Management Analyst
Health Services Research and
    Development
Veterans Administration-Northeast
    Region
West Roxbury, MA

I. THE ROLE OF QUALITY ASSURANCE IN THE PROFESSIONALIZATION OF THERAPEUTIC RECREATION

RAY WEST

Therapeutic Recreation began in hospitals because of the value of recreation for patients. Initially, services were provided in state and federal institutions specializing in long-term care for psychiatry, rehabilitation, or mental retardation. Our roots show that volunteers had much to do with the provision of recreation services in these hospital settings. We are all aware that in our early years there was considerable debate among our practitioners and with those from outside our profession about whether we were a "therapy" service or a part of the milieu, which had therapeutic value. In many, if not most, situations, we were expected to deliver recreation services as a part of the therapeutic milieu and for the most part, that probably is the type of service we delivered. We debated whether we were an allied health profession or more closely aligned with the recreation movement.

In the 1960's and '70's, we saw several significant developments which have had profound impact on the development of the therapeutic recreation profession. In the mid-1960's, the Medicare program and other legislation greatly expanded and developed the health-care industry in the United States (Reitter, 1985). As a society we were concerned about the welfare of our citizens; health care and, to a lesser degree, recreation became important

1

concerns. It was also in the mid-1960's that we saw the development of the National Therapeutic Recreation Society as a branch of the National Recreation and Park Association; a bold move to unite the recreation profession. Therapeutic recreation pursued several professionalization efforts, including, to name a few:

1. Discussion and debate about philosophy to help us understand our value and guide us in provision of services,
2. Expansion of our literature and our body of knowledge,
3. Development of standards to guide the delivery of therapeutic recreation service,
4. Expansion of our national registration program which certified practitioners,
5. Development of special recreation services for the ill, disabled, and handicapped.

(NTRS, 1978; Hunnicut, 1978)

The early 1970's saw continued growth of the profession and expansion of TR service into a variety of health-care and human-service settings, including community hospitals, community mental-health centers, nursing homes, community recreation settings, etc. At this time, health care and human services in the United States were continuing to expand. However, by the mid-1970's, we began to be concerned about the rapid increase in the cost of health care and human services. Measures were taken to control the cost of health care, hopefully without having negative impact on the quality of care or the quality of life of individuals with disabilities. Quality assurance, which has been in existence for many years, began to emerge as an important concern.

From the latter 1970's to the present, we've become a society experiencing a variety of trends and changes. According to one popular book, *Megatrends* (1982), we have and are experiencing:

1. A move from an industrial to an information society,
2. A move from forced technology to high-tech/high-touch,
3. A move from a national economy to a world economy,
4. A move from short-term to long-term focus in business, industry and government,
5. A move from centralization to decentralization in terms of organizational structures,
6. A move from institutional help to self-help,
7. A move from representative democracy to participatory democracy,
8. A move from hierarchies to networking,

9. A move from north to south,
10. A move from either/or to multiple options.

The health-care and human-service industries have been greatly affected by these and other societal trends. We have moved in society from an orientation toward the highest quality of health care available to all, regardless of cost, to at least an equal and maybe even a primary orientation toward costs and financing. Due to federal and state legislation, we are experiencing retrenchment and reduction to some degree, and a largely market-driven approach to health care and human services. These trends have had, and will continue to have, a significant impact on the therapeutic recreation profession. From those outside our profession, the demands on the therapeutic recreation profession for accountability are greater than ever before. People's understanding and expectations for therapeutic recreation have also changed. Many still do not know much about our service, but where our service is provided the expectations for quality are greater than ever before. In clinical settings—inpatient, out-patient, home health, long-term care and community health—where most therapeutic recreation services are found, the expectation is that we demonstrate that we contribute to the improved functioning and independence of our clients. To survive in clinical settings, we must be understood as reasonable and necessary treatment services, provided as an aspect of active treatment.

As of 1984, we now have two national organizations for therapeutic recreation. Professionalization efforts continue and include:

1. Discussion and debate about philosophy and definition,
2. Expansion of our literature and body of knowledge,
3. Development and compliance with standards,
4. Certifying practitioners,
5. Increasing emphasis on issues relevant in clinical settings, i.e., reimbursement, etc.

Hopefully a major reason for these and other professionalization efforts is to assure the quality of services provided. We must not lose sight of the reason our services developed—to be of assistance to the clients/consumers who want and need our help.

What does the future hold for TR? We can probably expect that the current health-care and human-service trends will continue to evolve and change the industry. A recent issue of *Hospital Management Review* (1986) described these changes:

> Because of over-capacity and declining utilization, the free-standing community hospital as we know it now will cease to exist by 1995.

To survive, hospitals will become integrated health care organizations (HCOs), providing a comprehensive range of services from acute care through nursing-home and home-health care. Payment will be in the form of capitated (per enrollee) rates. Virtually all physicians providing services in the HCO will be on a salary.

Chains of HCOs will be organized into health-care corporations (HCCs) owned by existing multi-hospital systems and insurance companies. Commercial insurance companies and Blue Cross will form HCOs by purchasing existing hospitals. It is predicted that, for all practical purposes, commercial health insurance as we know it will cease to exist by 1995. The distinction between insurer and provider will be gone.

What does this mean for us as a profession? It probably means that the market forces affecting health care and human services will continue to have significant impact on our profession. To survive, we have to demonstrate the efficacy of our service in these settings. We must measure the outcome of our service for the clients we serve and the service system of which we are a part. Quality assurance is a critically important focus for us today and it will be more important in the future. I believe that therapeutic recreation has much to contribute to health care and human services and that we can be one of the most innovative and valued health-care services of the future. Our individual and collective action as a profession is essential if we are to continue to evolve as a profession. We have a tremendous amount of professionalization to achieve in a short period of time if we are to succeed. Quality assurance has to be a primary and major focus. On behalf of the American Therapeutic Recreation Association (ATRA), I am pleased to be a part of this first professional conference on quality assurance and excited to know that those present today have chosen to accept this challenge. I encourage you to aggressively pursue the issue of quality assurance for therapeutic recreation over the next few days. I am confident that we can expand our knowledge and our professional horizons with the information which will be covered about quality assurance.

REFERENCES

Hospital Management Review. (1986). "Health Care Corporations (HCCs) to be Focal Point of Industry Competition in the 1990's." *5*(3), 4.

Hunnicut, B.K. (1978). "A Rejoinder to the Twelve-year History." *Therapeutic Recreation Journal, 12*(3), 15–19.

Naisbitt, J. (1982). *Megatrends.* New York, NY: Warner Books, Inc.

National Therapeutic Recreation Society. (1978). "NTRS: The First Twelve Years." *Therapeutic Recreation Journal, 12*(3), 4–14.

Reitter, M. (1986). *Pro's and Private Review: New Challenges for Therapeutic Recreation.* Unpublished manuscript. Chapel Hill, NC: University of North Carolina.

Reitter, M. (1986). *The History of Current Attempts to Reduce Health Care Costs.* Unpublished manuscript. Chapel Hill, NC: University of North Carolina.

ADDITIONAL RESOURCES

Compton, D.M. (1982). "Therapeutic Recreation at the Crossroads: Legislate, Advocate, or Abdicate." In G. Hitzhusen (Ed.), *Expanding Horizons in Therapeutic Recreation XI.* (pp. 6–15). Columbia, MO: University of Missouri.

Folkerth, J.E. (1983). "Status Report: State Section Update." *Therapeutic Recreation Journal, 1,* 7–11.

II. CONCEPTUAL BASIS OF QUALITY ASSURANCE: APPLICATION TO THERAPEUTIC RECREATION SERVICE

BOB RILEY

> We have granted the health professions access to the most secret and sensitive places in ourselves and entrusted to them matters that touch on our well-being, happiness and survival. In return, we have expected the professions to govern themselves so strictly that we need have no fear of exploitation or incompetence. (Donabedian, 1978, p. 111)

In light of this statement, to what extent have health professions lived up to this expectation of quality service? Addressing the same question more directly, to what degree does the therapeutic recreation profession assure quality service to its clientele? It would not be surprising to hear the response from most professionals that they inherently "feel" they provide quality-oriented services. However, when required to substantiate their claim, many would be left empty-handed, their answers lacking substance, and without much to show in evidence. The purpose of this paper is to address this concern. The concept of quality care will be explored and approaches available for measuring and monitoring such care will be outlined.

Quality Care

Quality of care has emerged as an important issue in health services because of its impact on the quality of life (Ullman, 1985). Several studies (Havel, 1981; Kahana, 1980; Langer & Rodin, 1976; Wolk & Telleen, 1976) have indicated a direct correlation between improved quality of service and the well-being of health-care recipients. But the impetus to design quality-assurance programs and to monitor their success is influenced by several other factors, many of which lie outside the control of the professional.

The emphasis on providing quality service stems directly from the critical issue of cost/benefit measurement in the health-care industry. Given skyrocketing costs, the necessity for accountability in health services becomes quite evident. The need for documentation of proven successes in respect to health-care services and techniques is vital. Within this environment of cost containment and capitation payment, it becomes essential that the best product be provided for the least amount of money spent.

In direct response to this impending crisis, accreditation has become of utmost importance in the health-care arena. Today, national regulatory organizations and local state-health agencies play a much more expanded role in the monitoring of health-care services. The concern for quality service today is directly linked to the preservation of health-care organizations in respect to their financial solvency as well as consumer satisfaction.

Ultimately, the underlying motivation for quality assurance should transcend the issues of financial accountability and program survivability. The desire to provide appropriate services and quality work should flourish from a sense of professional ethics. Being a professional and being part of a professional organization demands a sense of ethical commitment and the promotion of self-monitoring quality-assurance activities. As Kessner, et al (1973) have stated, "The question is no longer whether there will be intervention in health services to assure quality, but who will intervene and what methods they will use" (p. 189). The fact remains that if the profession (i.e., therapeutic recreation) does not employ effective quality-assurance mechanisms, then the health-care industry, accrediting organizations, and health-care regulatory agencies will. The danger in allowing this to occur lies in how *quality of care* will be defined and, of equal importance, how it will be measured.

Toward the Measurement of Quality Care. In attempting to focus upon a generally acceptable definition of quality care, it becomes quite apparent that this is not an easy task. The difficulty lies in the fact that "quality" has a multiplicity of meanings and is often used within varied contexts. Beyond the normative definition that the dictionary provides—*excellence; superiority; (Websters,* 1984)—"quality" is often defined simply within the context of "I know it when I see it," (Guaspari, 1985). This view of quality rests on the premise that one cannot explain it, but certainly we intuitively know it! The "goodness" approach to quality is, however, quickly eroding. In its place, emerging as a central focus of the business world today, is the view that "quality is conformance to requirements," (Crosby, 1984, p. 64). Through this regulatory approach, the definition of quality is determined by preset standards and accepted modes of measurement rather than by intrinsic characteristics. Thus this approach allows for quality to be viewed circuitously, in that as society's norms and values change and evolve, new standards and methods of measurement simultaneously emerge. The key, however, is in establishing mutually acceptable standards that constitute quality care.

Investigating the correlates to quality of care reveals that no national studies exist from which to obtain "an undistorted picture of the level and distribution of quality" (Donabedian, 1985a, p. 283). Donabedian, in addressing the epidemiology of quality, extracted information from various sources and found that "the distribution of behaviors that directly or indirectly connote quality reveals an astounding degree of variability among geographic areas, practitioners and institutions" (1985, p. 283). A consensus as to what constitutes quality of care varies significantly within the general care community (Marshik et al, 1983; Tash & Staher, 1982). Contrary to the business world's orientation to quality assurance (quality control and zero-production deficits), the health-care system involves a multitude of factors, including the human condition, which alters the simplicity of merely eliminating the negative aspects of production and building upon the positive attributes. As Russel Roth, former president of the American Medical Association, has stated:

> . . . good quality in medical care is not something which can be
> expressed in dollars of costs, hours of time or for that matter in
> decibels of political oratory. Quality of such medical care is not a
> tangible, qualifiable thing. (Jonas, 1981, p. 399).

In recent years, however, progress has been made in identifying key elements which contribute to a definition of quality health care. According to Graham (1982),

> The definition of quality encompasses both the technical, scien-
> tific aspect and the "art" of the care. The art of care refers to the
> manner in which physicians conduct themselves in relation to
> their patients (p. 9).

9

Donabedian (1985) expands the parameters of this conceptual framework and outlines the basic elements of the definition of quality care as follows:

Technical/Scientific: addresses balance between risks and benefits, and perceives quality health care in the following manner:

1. Promotion
2. Preservation
3. Restoration

Interpretational/Art: meeting socially defined values and norms given individual or social ethics. Quality care is perceived as:

1. Acceptable
2. Pleasing
3. Rewarding

Amenities/Environmental: providing added fixtures (TV, clean room, phone, etc.) which increase patient satisfaction and promote quality care via:

1. Comfort
2. Individuality
3. Security

Given these basic elements, the definition of quality care still remains difficult to pinpoint, depending upon the perspective of the definer. Consumers, practitioners, administrators, and society at large place varied and conflicting degrees of emphasis upon each of these broadly defined elements of care. The "Art vs. Science" literature (Sussman et al, 1967; Sanazaro & Williamson, 1968; Price et al, 1972; Smith & Mentzner, 1970) indicates that in terms of the definition of quality care, a substantial gap exists between the practitioner and consumer. In discussing the validation (acceptance) process involving an operational definition of quality of care, Donabedian (1980) identifies three distinct views:

1) *Absolutist:* practitioner-oriented; stresses technical aspects and ignores cost.

2) *Individualized:* consumer-oriented; measures technical care and amenities, accepts costs based upon an individual cost/benefit ratio.

3) *Social:* business/political-oriented; measures technical care via effectiveness, bases costs upon capitation or prospective payment.

In a broad sense, it can be stated that the "absolutist" perspective operationalizes health care from a maximum effort perspective; the "individualized" perspective supports choice along the continuum of adequate—optimal—maximum effort, depending upon the cost/outcome ratio; and the "social" proponent supports adequate care, in the most efficient manner, in an effort to depreciate costs.

In a general sense, it can be stated that consumers desire equal emphasis on technical as well as interpersonal care due to the fact that these two elements are so interdependent. However, the social view perceives quality care as being assessed by monetary measures that merely insure adequate care within a minimum range of options. This conflict places the practitioner in a rather precarious situation.

In summary, the definition of quality care should be viewed within a contextual framework that takes into account perspective, values, and purpose. (See Figure 2.1.) The very nature of quality is that it is dynamic and ever changing. As knowledge, values, and resources evolve, so, too, does the view of what constitutes quality of care (Graham, 1982). Once quality has been defined within a given situational context, the next challenge is to develop a strategic process to assure its presence within therapeutic care environments.

Figure 2.1   Contextual Influences on the Definition of Quality

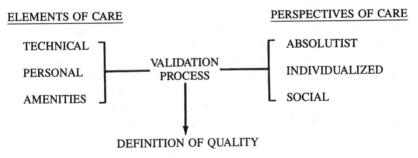

ELEMENTS OF CARE   PERSPECTIVES OF CARE

TECHNICAL   ABSOLUTIST
                          VALIDATION
PERSONAL   PROCESS   INDIVIDUALIZED

AMENITIES   SOCIAL

DEFINITION OF QUALITY

Quality Assurance

Quality Assurance (QA) is a process that enables the health professional to identify areas of improvement, detect potential problem areas, and design strategies for overcoming deficient areas in patient care (JCAH, 1984). The evolution of QA has been a dynamic process, with significant shifts in philosophy, concept, strategy, and evaluation occurring during the last five decades. Today QA is defined in a multiplicity of ways ranging from evaluation (Bull, 1985) to management (Reynolds & O'Morrow, 1985) to process (Pena et al, 1984). In light of the acceptance of the definition of quality care as conformance to standards, the Pena et al (1984) definition of QA is most pragmatic. These authors define QA as:

> . . . a process that sets the standards for performance, provides information about the achievement of those standards, and monitors whether improvement has taken place and whether the standards are being met. (p. XIV)

A review of health-care literature reveals a plethora of information regarding the QA process. A synthesis of the basic elements comprising the quality-assurance process is as follows:

—Program Planning
—Set Standards
—Systematic Monitoring of Routine Behavior
—Comprehensive Design
—Evaluation of Recognized Deficiencies
—Recommendations for Alternative Methods
—Establishment of Mechanisms for Adopting Recommendations

In essence, QA is implemented to assure that standards of acceptable professional behavior are met. Thus the driving force behind QA activities should be professional standards instead of regulatory and accrediting organizations. According to the Joint Commission on Accreditation of Hospitals (JCAH), the QA process must be implemented through the utilization of written criteria. Furthermore, the responsibility for the establishment of such measurements lies chiefly with specific service departments in coordination with their respective professional-affiliated organizations (JCAH, 1984). This process of assuring quality professional behavior occurs within two distinct domains: Global QA and Programmatic QA.

Global Quality Assurance

Global QA is the utilization of control mechanisms by professional organizations in order to assure quality professional behavior by their members. These procedures are referred to as global because they uniformly address the behavior of individuals throughout the profession. Specifically, global QA activities assure: 1) the quality of service rendered, 2) the appropriateness of service rendered, and 3) the level of competence and skill demonstrated by professional members. A schematic illustration depicting global QA activities and their relationship to professional behavior is provided in Figure 2.2. Also represented within the global QA configuration is the circuitous nature of the QA process, illustrating the continuous monitoring/ feedback loop which allows for growth and change at both the professional/ organization level as well as at the individual/professional level.

Among the six global QA activities listed in Figure 2.2, standards of practice are deemed the most critical. Standards of practice determine the protocols of service and thus establish the basis for professional behavior. In addition, standards of practice also serve as the blueprint for the establishment of programmatic QA procedures.

Figure 2.2 Global Quality Assurance

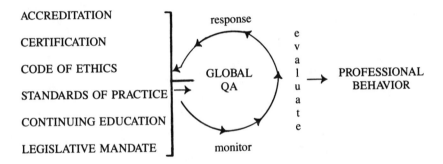

Literature on the subject of QA and standards of practice in relationship to therapeutic recreation is minimal, and has not kept pace with the rapidly evolving issue of quality patient care. As Navar and Dunn (1981) have pointed out: "an accurate 'state of the art' description of therapeutic recreation quality assurance involvement is still unknown" (p. 2). Other authors place it at a level of "frustration" (Reynolds & O'Morrow, 1985, p. 107).

Although therapeutic recreation standards of practice have been established by the National Therapeutic Recreation Society (NTRS, 1980), there still exist, as with many other professional services, doubts as to whether such standards truly assure quality of care (Drude & Nelson, 1982). Constant monitoring and evaluation in this area are needed to assist professionals in identifying the "critical elements" of the therapeutic-recreation treatment model and to establish acceptable measures toward validating such elements of patient care. The measurement of appropriate standards of practice occurs at the client interaction level under the auspices of programmatic quality assurance.

Programmatic Quality Assurance

Programmatic QA (Figure 2.3) is a process utilized by health-care organizations and/or professional service departments to assure quality care at the specific professional/client interaction level. The major approaches in use within the health-care field today are hospital-staff review committees, professional review organizations (PROs), distinct measures of patient satisfactions, and departmental quality-assurance programs (Jonas, 1981). The importance of programmatic quality assurance is well documented (Vangunas, 1979; Vangunas et al, 1979; Reeder, 1981; Tan, 1978; Ward, 1984), as evidenced by the fact that most accrediting agencies (i.e., Joint Commission on Accreditation of Hospitals) require it as a necessary component for organization accreditation.

Figure 2.3 Programmatic Quality Assurance

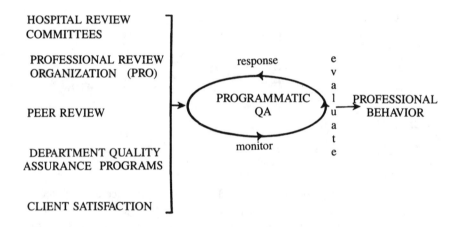

Ideally, a feedback loop exists between programmatic QA and global QA. The routine monitoring and evaluation at the service level provides an accurate measurement reflecting whether standards of practice (established globally at professional levels) truly assure quality performance.

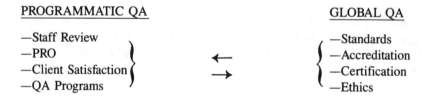

PROGRAMMATIC QA

—Staff Review
—PRO
—Client Satisfaction
—QA Programs

GLOBAL QA

—Standards
—Accreditation
—Certification
—Ethics

14

Quality Assurance Feedback System

The systematic approach to assuring quality professional behavior is, of course, not as simplistic as it appears. The process involves the commitment of both practitioners and professional organizations. Specific methodologies for coordinating such a process must be established and implemented if the system is to be of value. Presently, no such effort is being supported within the field of therapeutic recreation.

Quality Assessment in Programmatic Quality Assurance. At the specific client/provider interaction level, quality assurance is implemented to ascertain the level of quality care. According to Graham (1982):

> Quality assessment is the process of establishing the effectiveness of some aspect of health care in order to develop a foundation for current or future decision-making. Quality assurance includes the implementation of the quality assessment findings (p. XIII).

Delimiting this process one step further, quality monitoring is identified as the surveillance sub-element of quality assessment. Quality monitoring is the data-collection phase of quality assessment, and is viewed as an ongoing and systematic process. Graphically, the process is as follows:

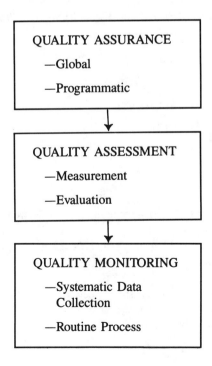

15

The process of quality assessment employs a multitude of methodologies and approaches. Review of the QA literature reveals a variety of schemata representing numerous techniques for evaluating and monitoring quality of care (Brook, 1973; Donabedian, 1966, 1968, 1980, 1982, 1985; Sanazaro & Williamson, 1968). A basic review of these approaches reveals the presence of four major levels of development. These developmental levels are standards of practice, approaches to evaluation, criteria, and criteria formation (see Figure 2.4).

Figure 2.4 Assessment of Quality Care

I. QUALITY CARE BASED UPON *STANDARDS OF PRACTICE:*
- NORMATIVE
- EMPIRICAL

II. *APPROACHES* TO QUALITY CARE MEASUREMENT:
- STRUCTURE
- PROCESS
- OUTCOME

III. *CRITERIA* APPLIED TO MEASUREMENT APPROACHES:
- EXPLICIT
- IMPLICIT

IV. FORMATION OF *CRITERIA:*
- ELEMENTS
- INDICATORS
- CRITERIA

Standards of Practice: As previously stated, standards of practice serve as the foundation for quality assessment. Standards, regardless of whether they are at a macro level (professional organization) or a micro level (departmental service plan), establish the protocols for professional behavior. According to Reynolds and O'Morrow (1985):

> . . . it is not so much a question of developing and implementing standards along with having the standards accepted by administrators and accrediting bodies, but more whether the standards assure quality (p. 104).

At the present time, there is a scarcity of data available that begins to address this concern. The status of therapeutic recreation standards (NTRS, 1980; Van Andel, 1981), is that they are extremely broad and in some respects philosophically disjointed as to the profession's mission statement. However, these standards represent a good start and a concrete example of the type of work that needs to be initiated toward assuring quality service within therapeutic recreation.

Standards of practice are established via several different procedures and are essentially derived from either "empirical" standards, "normative" standards, or, in some circumstances, both (Donabedian, 1984). Empirical standards represent actual practice and have been validated through research. These standards, when applied, represent a minimum level of performance or tolerance with respect to professional practice. A major drawback of empirical standards, according to Reynolds and O'Morrow (1985),

> is that service may appear to be adequate in comparison to that in other settings and yet fall short of what is attainable through the full application of current therapeutic recreation knowledge and practice (p. 105).

Normative standards, in contrast, represent desired rather than the observed performance (Donabedian, 1982). Such standards are derived from previously documented sources (i.e., textbooks) or from consensus feedback reflecting professional expert opinion. The standard can be set at any level, depending upon the desired level of quality to be attained. In respect to normative standards, levels of tolerance are usually set quite high. The merit of utilizing the normative approach to formulate standards of practice is that there exists a closer relationship between what is being measured and what is considered indicative of quality service.

Regardless of the derivation of standards utilized in therapeutic recreation practice, continuous testing and assessment must be implemented to assure the validity of such standards.

Approaches to Quality Care Measurement

It is generally recognized that Donabedian (1968, 1980, 1982) has developed a universally accepted classification of approaches to quality assessment. This classification system views quality measurement as occurring within three distinct domains: structure, process, and outcome (see Figure 2.5).

The most commonly used approach toward measuring quality of service is that of structure. Structure appraisal involves the measurement of various features of the care environment. Aspects of service such as qualification of

Figure 2.5 Approaches to Quality Assessment

- STRUCTURE EVALUATION

    —PHYSICAL FACILITIES

    —RESOURCES

    —ORGANIZATIONAL ELEMENTS

- PROCESS EVALUATION

    —PRACTITIONER/CLIENT INTERACTION

    —ACTIVITIES THAT CONSTITUTE CARE

- OUTCOME EVALUATION

    —EFFECTS OF CARE

    —END RESULTS

    —CONSEQUENCES TO HEALTH

Donabedian, 1982

staff, financial resources, equipment, location, physical appearance, and operation of program are evaluated, usually from a normative level.

Structure, at best, is regarded as an assurance criteria and not an assessment criteria (Donabedian, 1980). Structure evaluation reveals only general tendencies and relates to quality service on an assumptive basis; that is, if certain structural variables are present, then it is assumed that quality of care exists. However, an insufficient number of studies substantiate that structure variables increase quality performance (Jonas, 1981). However, this does not condemn the use of structural assessment entirely. It has been suggested that structure evaluation be utilized only in the absence of the more valid process-and-outcome approaches (Donabedian, 1982).

Process evaluation involves measurement of the actual practice of the therapeutic recreation service. Therefore, process evaluation is more indicative of quality assessment in comparison to structure evaluation. Process appraisal measures the behavior of the therapeutic recreation professional in respect to the established standards of care (standards of practice). Aspects of professional service that are measured, for example, are: completed assessment, written program objectives, proper data collection and documentation, and discharge summary. The major assumption is that such practices are inherently good for the client and, furthermore, that process procedures lead to expected desirable outcomes.

18

In critique, most process standards are normatively derived and tend to stress optimum or maximum levels of care. They also tend to ignore the interpersonal aspects of care—the art of care—because such standards are professionally oriented and based upon an absolutist perspective.

The assessment of outcomes in the quality-assessment process focuses upon the evaluation of end results. Outcome assessment monitors the changes in health status and patient behavior, as well as patient satisfaction. Outcome variables are tested via precise measurement and often possess a high level of causal validity in reference to acceptable norms of quality care. Another positive attribute of outcome measurement is the direct involvement of the patient in contributing to what is deemed and accepted as quality service.

Unfortunately, due to the rigorous nature of outcome measurement, evaluation is often time-consuming and costly. Additionally, determining causality of desired outcomes of quality care is often difficult to accomplish. While it may be determined that desired outcomes of care have been realized, there is often no evidence that the professional practices that brought about such results were of a quality nature.

Approaches to measurement of quality care have been summarized as follows:

> The structural approach examines the setting of care; the process approach examines what goes on between the provider(s) and the patient; the outcome approach examines the results of the encounter or lack thereof between the patient and the health care delivery system (Jonas, 1981, p. 403).

Thus the choice of measurement approach is a situational decision; structural techniques are often used in the global QA process while programmatic QA utilizes process and outcome techniques.

Ideally, the utilization of a combined approach is most effective, as exemplified by the "tracer method" (Kessner et al, 1973). This method combines both process and outcome measurement in an effort to establish a causal relationship between desired outcomes and antecedents to quality care. QA programs and research efforts utilizing this method of measurement are virtually non-existent in the field of therapeutic recreation. However, they are greatly needed.

Formation of Criteria

Within all three approaches to the measurement of quality care, criteria are used as part of the evaluation process. In a broad sense, criteria can be viewed as being *implicit* or *explicit* in nature. Implicit criteria exist in the mind of the evaluator. Measurement involving implicit criteria is considered subjective and relies upon the evaluator's perception of what are acceptable and non-acceptable levels of practice. Evaluators are selected based upon their training, levels of expertise, and individual performance records. It is assumed that competent professionals will be able to recognize "good practice" and thus are qualified to judge the quality of care provided.

Explicit criteria, conversely, are pre-established indicators of quality care. They are derived from an empirical process of a consensus agreement and exist in written form. The formation of explicit criteria involves the development of *elements, indicators,* and *criteria standards.*

Elements constitute the various aspects of care or service to be assessed. Indicators establish the general acceptable norms or levels at which such elements of service should be rendered, while criteria designate specific upper and/or lower limits of acceptable practice. Often indicators and criteria are combined in an attempt to facilitate measurement. Together, indicators and criteria establish the general rule of goodness to be followed and also set the precise statistical count of what constitutes adequate, optimum, and maximum levels of care. An example of explicit criteria in relationship to therapeutic recreation practice would be as follows:

ELEMENT: Leisure Functioning

INDICATOR: Increase in Independent Leisure Functioning

CRITERION   Preset Number of Self-Directed Activities
STANDARD: Attempted During One Week

This illustration is an example of an outcome measurement that uses the leisure functioning element as the segment of service to be monitored. The indicator, in relationship to this element, is that increased, independent functioning is desirable. The outcome measurement of whether adequate-optimal-maximal care has been provided would be determined by the criterion standard, which was pre-set prior to measurement.

In summary, quality assessment involves two types of standards, three approaches to evaluation, two categories of criteria, and three substeps to explicit criteria. Most critical to the process of quality assessment is the establishment of elements of service. In many respects, selected elements of service serve as the underpinnings of the standards of practice. Evaluation of such elements provides an empirical foundation for normatively derived standards of practice, and in essence supports or refutes their validity. Such evaluation should be accomplished at both the organizational and departmental level, as well as on a national level. The examination of therapeutic recreation standards and elements of care is critical to the issue of quality assurance as well as to the advancement of the therapeutic recreation profession. As Reynolds and O'Morrow (1985) have urged:

> Therapeutic recreation has shown extraordinary adaptive capacities, but to continue to do so will require further research into standards of practice so as to ensure quality assurance. The practical task of establishing reliability and validity in our standards is formidable, but it must be done (p. 108).

Further Thoughts on Quality Assurance

Simply stated, QA is not a flash-in-the-pan idea that will dissipate as quickly as it appears to have emerged. QA has been discussed in various health-care circles for decades. Even if the present health-care financial picture becomes more focused, quality of patient care will undoubtedly remain a central theme.

Therapeutic recreation professionals need to address the QA process with more zeal and conviction. Practitioners need to establish operational definitions of quality assessment within their therapeutic recreation service plans. Additionally, professionals need to advocate their QA findings to hospital administrators and service chiefs in an effort to illustrate therapeutic recreation's contribution to quality health care.

Nationally, in a collective effort, therapeutic recreation professionals need to systematically evaluate their standards of practice and test them accordingly for empirical validity. Such efforts would create more appropriate structural standards (global QA) as well as ensure the utilization of process and outcome measures. Currently there exists a gap between practitioners and academic researchers in respect to how quality care is measured and how it can be assured (Jonas, 1981, p. 429). Researchers tend to reject structural indicators as ineffective, but practitioner and professional organizations continue to support such indicators in their certification, accreditation, and licensing practices. This conflict in professional direction needs to be addressed and rectified if the therapeutic recreation profession is going to make progress toward accountability in the general health-care arena.

The future of therapeutic recreation will be determined by the success of professional efforts to substantiate the claim that it contributes to the overall well-being of health-care consumers. Quality assurance and quality assessment are proven processes that can assist in this endeavor. The challenge of establishing the QA process in therapeutic recreational services is a formidable task, but based upon ethical concern and professional advancement, it must be addressed.

REFERENCES

Brook, R.H. (1973). *Quality of Care Assessment: A Comparison of Five Methods of Peer Review.* National Center for Health Services Research and Development. Washington, D.C.: USDHEW.

Bull, M. (1985). "Quality Assurance: Its Origins, Transformations, and Prospects." In Meisenheimer, C.G., (Ed.), *Quality Assurance.* Rockville, MD: Aspen Systems Corp.

Crosby, P. (1984). *Quality without Tears.* NY: New American Library.

Donabedian, A. (1985). *Explorations in Quality Assessment and Monitoring, Volume III: The Methods and Findings of Quality Assessment and Monitoring.* Ann Arbor, MI: Health Administration Press.

Donabedian, A. (1985a). "The Epidemiology of Quality." *Inquiry.* 22.

Donabedian, A. (1982). *Explorations in Quality Assessment and Monitoring, Volume II: The Criteria and Standards of Quality.* Ann Arbor, MI: Health Administration Press.

Donabedian, A. (1980). *Explorations in Quality Assessment and Monitoring, Volume I: The Definition of Quality and Approaches to Its Assessment.* Ann Arbor, MI: Health Administration Press.

Donabedian, A. (1978). "The Quality of Medical Care." *Science, 200* (May 26), 856–864.

Donabedian, A. (1968). "Promoting Quality Through Evaluating the Process of Patient Care." *Medical Care, 6.*

Donabedian, A. (1966). "Evaluating the Quality of Medical Care." *Milbank Memorial Fund Quarterly, 44.*

Drude, K. & Nelson, R. (1982). "Quality Assurance: A Challenge for Community Mental Health Centers." *Professional Psychology, 13*(1), 85–90.

Graham, N. (1982). *Quality Assurance in Hospitals.* Rockville, MD: Aspen Publications.

Guaspari, J. (1985). *I Know It When I See It: A Modern Fable About Quality.* New York: American Management Association.

Havel, Z. (1981). "Quality of Care, Congruence, and Well-being among Institutionalized Aged." *Gerontologist, 21* 523–531.

Joint Commission on Accreditation of Hospitals. (1984). *Quality and Appropriateness Review.* JCAH Audiocassette series.

Jonas, S. (1981). *Health Care Delivery in the United States.* NY: Springer Publishing.

Kahana, E. (1980). "Alternative Models of Personal Environment Fit: Prediction of Morale in Three Homes for the Aged." *Journal of Gerontology, 35,* 584–595.

Kessner, D.M. et al. (1973). "Assessing Health Quality—the Case for Tracers." *New England Journal of Medicine, 288,* 189.

Langer, E. & Rodin, I. (1976). "The Effects of Choice and Enhanced Personal Responsibility: A Field Experiment in an Institutional Setting." *Journal of Personality and Social Psychology, 34,* 191–198.

Marshik, J. et al (1983). "Planning Is the Key to Successful QA Programs." *Hospitals, 55*(11), 67–73.

National Therapeutic Recreation Society. (1980). *Standards of Practice for Therapeutic Recreation Service.* Alexandria, VA: NRPA.

Navar, N. & Dunn, J. (Eds.) (1981). *Quality Assurance: Concerns for Therapeutic Recreation.* Urbana-Champaign, IL: University of Illinois.

Pena, J. et al. (1984). *Hospital Quality Assurance.* Rockville, MD: Aspen Systems Corp.

Price, P. et al. (1972). *Measurement and Predictors of Physician Performance: Two Decades of Intermittently Sustained Research.* Salt Lake City, UT: University of Utah.

Reeder, M. (1981). "The Benefits of Areawide Quality Review." *Quality Review Bulletin,* December 2–3.

Reynolds, R. & O'Morrow, G. (1985). *Problems, Issues and Concepts in Therapeutic Recreation.* Englewood Cliffs, NJ: Prentice Hall, Inc.

Sanazaro, P. & Williamson, J. (1968). "A Classification of Physician Performance in Internal Medicine." *Journal of Medical Education, 43* (March).

Smith, D. & Mentzner, C. (1970). "Differential Perceptions of Health Care Quality in a Prepaid Group Practice." *Medical Care, 8* (July–August).

Sussman, M., et al (1967). *The Walking Patient: A Study in Outpatient Care.* Cleveland, OH: The Press of Western Reserve University.

Tan, M.W. (1978). "Problem Areas in Multidisciplinary Audit." *Quality Review Bulletin,* November, 33–35.

Tash, W., & Staher, G. (1982). "Enhancing the Utilization of Evaluation Findings." *Community Mental Health Journal, 18*(3), 180–189.

Ullmann, S. (1985). "The Impact of Quality on Cost in the Provision of Long-term Care." *Inquiry, 22* (Fall), 282–292.

Vangunas, A., Egelston, M., Hopkins, J. & Walczak, R. (1979). "Principles of Quality Assurance." *QRB,* February, 3–6.

Vangunas, A. (1979). "Quality Assessment: Alternate Alternatives." *QRB,* February, 7–10.

Ward, M. (1984). "An Annotated Bibliography: Quality Assurance Background, Theory and Perspectives." *Quality Review Bulletin,* August, 248–250.

Webster's New World Dictionary, 2nd ed. (1984). Cleveland, OH: The World Publishing Company.

Wolk, S. & Telleen, S. (1976). "Psychological and Social Correlates of Life Satisfaction as a Function of Residential Constraint." *Journal of Gerontology, 31,* 89–98.

III. YOU WANT ME TO DO WHAT? REGULATORY STANDARDS IN THERAPEUTIC RECREATION

GEORGE DONOVAN

The 1980's have been an era of accountability and cost effectiveness in the health-care provider field. We have seen an increased emphasis on quality assurance (QA) and the development and implementation of new resource allocation methodologies: diagnostic related groups (DRGs) and resource utilization groups (RUGs). These new methodologies and the increased emphasis on quality assurance have placed a heavy burden on the therapeutic recreation professional, who must keep abreast of this evolutionary process and incorporate these changes in order to provide state-of-the-art services to clients. Similarly, the regulatory agencies (i.e., JCAH) that accredit health-care facilities are also striving to meet the needs of an ever-changing health-care environment. To ensure that the voluntary accreditation process remains a viable force for assuring quality in health-care facilities, the Joint Commission on Accreditation of Hospitals conducts its accreditation process with attention to changing practices in health care and current trends in the health-care delivery system (LaBrenz, 1985, p. 1). Therapeutic recreation professionals must also continue to be sensitive to health-care changes.

This article describes a state-of-the-art quality-assurance program which includes the role of regulatory agencies, internal and external review strategies, and an illustration and interpretation of quality-care standards. The

25

agenda will include an overview of each regulatory agency, including JCAH, the Commission on Accreditation of Rehabilitation Facilities (CARF), the Health Care Financing Administration (HCFA), the National Therapeutic Recreation Society (NTRA), and the Systematic External Review Process (SERP).

Standards. It is impossible to determine the quality of therapeutic recreation services without an understanding of the use and interrelationship of standards. Standards are predetermined elements against which aspects of quality treatment can be compared (Waterman, Johnson, and Cantrell, 1981, p. 127). When applying appropriate standards, therapeutic recreation professionals must remember that they are general in nature, and that utilizing them is like attempting to bake a cake with a written recipe that contains the ingredients but not the specific amounts of each. Because of the growing variety of health-care settings, standards that are more general and less prescriptive allow each individual facility to develop programs that will suit their unique needs (LaBrenz, 1981, p. 5). Professionals must be able to apply these to their specific programs, allowing them to serve "as a set of guidelines representing the best thinking of those involved in services for the people with disabilities (CARF, 1986, p. 3). CARF also believes that standards are "an excellent management tool and a blueprint for organizational planning." The therapeutic recreation professional must be able to utilize this blueprint and apply state-of-the-art services in order to be proactive with the ever-changing health-care system.

Many sources of standards currently exist for therapeutic recreation: the *Personnel and Agency Standards* developed by Doris Berryman, the *NTRS Standards of Practice, JCAH Standards, CARF Standards,* and *HCFA Standards.* Each of these will be discussed below in order to show how their recommendations can be utilized to generate more specific agency standards.

Overview of Standards. The standards instrument developed by Berryman (Johnson, et al, 1984) is a classic document to be studied before developing any agency standards. This comprehensive checklist describes fifty-five different standards and 214 different criteria within them. It covers such areas as philosophies and goals, personnel considerations, programming, facilities and equipment, and evaluation and research.

The National Therapeutic Recreation Society published its *Standards of Practice* in 1980. This document, along with the *NTRS Guidelines for Administration of Therapeutic Recreation Service in Clinical and Residential Facilities* (1980), was derived from Berryman's work, and professionals must be aware and utilize these available resources when developing agency standards. Specifically stated, the *NTRS Standards of Practice,* published in 1980, provides for the following:

1. Comprehensive Services Available:
   A. Clinical
   B. Leisure Education
   C. General Recreation
2. Objectives Written
3. Individual Treatment Plans
4. Medical Record Documentation
5. Specific Times Alloted for Therapeutic Recreation
6. Ethical Practices

What is most revealing here is that even our professional organization is very general in its outline for *Standards of Practice.* However, we must keep in mind that "standards are only minimal to assure minimal quality of service." (Waterman, Johnson, Cantrell,, 1981, p. 139).

The JCAH has published five sets of standards: the *Accreditation Manual for Hospitals* (1980); the *Consolidated Standards Manual for Child, Adolescent and Adult Psychology, Alcoholism and Drug Abuse Facilities and Facilities Serving the Mentally Retarded/Developmentally Disabled* (1985); the *Long Term Care Standards Manual* (1986); the *Hospice Standards Manual* (1983); and the *Ambulatory Health Care Standards Manual* (1986).

Each standards manual contains a section on general administrative policies and procedures that lists the eligibility criteria for determining who may apply for a JCAH survey. This section also describes the process by which JCAH surveys and accredits a facility (LaBrenz, 1985, p. 7).

Three of the JCAH standards manuals specifically contain therapeutic recreation standards. They are Chapter Ten in the *Long Term Care Standards Manual,* Chapter Thirty in the *Consolidated Standards Manual,* and Chapter Nineteen in the *Accreditation Manual for Hospitals.* However, when developing agency and/or departmental standards, professionals must be aware that other chapters in these manuals have standards relating to therapeutic recreation, including those on quality assurance, patient care monitoring, staff growth and development, and assessment.

Consolidated Standards (1985) includes therapeutic recreation in a section on activities services. Chapter Thirty, "Rehabilitation Services," in this section includes the following guidelines:

1. Provide activity services.
2. Have a written plan for organization.
3. Plan on using community resources.
4. Write down goals and objectives.

5. Write down policies and procedures.
6. Plan activities throughout the week.
7. Document medical records.
8. Give patients leisure time.
9. Do not label vehicles.
10. Hire a qualified supervisor.
11. Hire sufficient staff.
12. Review goals, objectives, and roles.
13. Keep statistical records.
14. Plan a staff development program.
15. Be active in committees and conferences.
16. Be trained for emergencies.
17. Encourage studies, evaluation, and research.
18. Have sufficient space, equipment, and facilities.
19. Ensure quality and appropriateness of patient care.
20. Continuously monitor important aspects of care.
21. Give a periodic assessment of monitors.
22. Document findings.
23. Make sure your activities QA program is part of a facility QA program.

The second set of JCAH Standards that cover therapeutic recreation are provided in the *Long Term Care Standards Manual* published in 1986. The chapter on "Patient/Resident Activities" describes four standards based on a principle whose clear intent is that you assess needs and develop individual programs based on these needs (Johnson, Donovan, Bellah, Waterman, 1984, p. 58). The JCAH *Long Term Care Standards Manual*, published in 1986, provides the following suggestions in Chapter Ten:

1. Organize and staff to actively meet needs of patients/residents.
2. Make the staff responsible for developing, documenting, and maintaining activities.
3. Hire a qualified patient-activities coordinator.
4. Hire a sufficient staff.
5. Acquire suitable activity space.
6. Acquire suitable supplies and equipment.
7. Organize activities suited to needs.
8. Offer a variety of activities.
9. Make an activities schedule available.
10. Offer independent activities.
11. Create assessment areas.
12. Monitor quality and appropriateness of activities.

The third and final JCAH standards manual that contains guidelines on therapeutic recreation is the *Accreditation Manual for Hospitals,* published in

1986. Chapter Nineteen, "Rehabilitation Services," includes six standards under the Recreational Therapy Section. These cover the following areas:

1. Development, maintenance, and expression of appropriate leisure/social lifestyles,
2. Assessment of patient's leisure,
3. Treatment programs,
4. Leisure Education programs,
5. Goal achievement monitoring.

Professionals need to be aware of the above JCAH standards, along with those of other regulatory agencies that department services must observe (Waterman, 1986, p. 5).

The Commission on Accreditation of Rehabilitation Facilities (CARF) has published a *Standards Manual for Organizations Serving People with Disabilities* in 1986. CARF Standards are for individual programs or services in the following areas:

> Comprehensive inpatient rehabilitation
> Spinal cord injury programs
> Chronic pain management programs
> Brain injury programs
> Outpatient medical rehabilitation
> Infant and early childhood development programs
> Vocational evaluation
> Work adjustment
> Programs in industry
> Occupational skills training
> Job placement
> Work services
> Activity services
> Residential services
> Respite services
> Independent living programs
> Alcoholism and drug-abuse treatment programs
> Psychosocial programs

Therapeutic recreation is specifically mentioned in the CARF Standards for comprehensive in-patient rehabilitation, spinal-cord injury programs, chronic pain management programs, brain injury programs, and outpatient medical rehabilitation. CARF, like JCAH, also has a chapter devoted to activity services; however, unlike JCAH it includes standards not related to therapeutic recreation (i.e., allergies, hospital preferred, designation of primary physician, etc.). The CARF manual presents additional regulatory areas that therapeutic recreation professionals must be aware of in order to provide quality services. These include intake and orientation, assessment and individual program planning, program management, treatment and training, referral, discharge and follow-up, and case records, to name a few. The CARF manual, like the JCAH, is a functional manual. Professionals must be aware of this so that those functional areas that have been previously mentioned can be applied to the therapeutic recreation services. CARF Activity services standards provide for the following:

1. Lists of activity resources and capabilities,
2. Curricula and course outlines for areas of instruction,
3. Individual case records,
4. Written grievance and appeal procedures,
5. Minutes of meetings of those served and management.

Also under the residential services standards of CARF, a daily activities schedule standard provides for free time, (thirty hours of activities provided outside the home), integrated with the community and documented with evidence of client choice.

The final regulatory agency that provides standards for the therapeutic recreation profession is the Health Care Finance Administration (HCFA). (See *Federal Register* no. 42 subpart J, 1976.) HCFA is an agency under the Department of Health and Human Services whose standards were developed for the reimbursement of Medicare funds. Therefore the HCFA standards are different from those of JCAH and CARF in that they are mandated under public law, while the aforementioned standards are all voluntary procedures. As stated in the "HCFA Medicare and Medicaid Guidelines" (*Federal Register*, 1976, p. 236): "A provider of health services is not entitled to participate in the Medicare program until it has submitted a participation agreement to the Secretary of Health and Human Services and the Secretary has approved the agreement. In addition, the provider must be in compliance with the provisions of Title VI of the Civil Rights Act." The providers of HCFA services also must participate in Utilization Reviews and Professional Standards Review Organizations (PSRO's) in order to assure quality care to patients.

The HCFA standards are published in the *Federal Register* by the Government Printing Office. Unlike JCAH or CARF, they do not have specific manuals. Because these changes are a result of public law, HCFA uses the *Federal Register* publication to announce changes. HCFA standards have many classifications similar to those of JCAH and CARF (i.e., governing body, physical environment, medical staff, nursing, dietary department, medical record department, pharmacy or drug room, laboratories, radiology department, medical library, complementing departments, etc.).

The only specific mention of the therapeutic recreation profession in the HCFA standards is under the section "Special Rules and Exceptions Applying to Psychiatric and Tuberculosis Hospitals." This section provides for therapeutic recreation services through the following procedures:

1. Treatment is documented with such frequency to assure active therapeutic effort.
2. The individual's capacity to manage activities is maintained or increased.
3. Staff provides for social interaction.
4. A qualified staff is retained.
5. Sufficient staff is retained.
6. Qualified supervision is provided. (p. 238, 1976)

Also in this section, HCFA standards suggest the following:

1. Diversionary and recreation services
2. An adjunct to the active treatment program
3. Registered OT direction
4. Qualified supervision of assistants, aides, or volunteers (p. 392, 1976)

Therapeutic recreation professionals providing services under the HCFA Standards must be aware of how these specific standards are related to their field. However, they must also realize that other HCFA Standards areas are directly related to therapeutic recreation services (i.e., medical records, utilization reviews, discharge summaries, and special staff requirements).

Agency Standards. As you can see, there are many standards available to therapeutic recreation professionals for developing agency standards. These should guide them in the implementation and provision of services. As Waterman (1986) states: "When developing Standards, your service must be in compliance with all Standards that have regulatory authority over you. Furthermore, they should reflect the philosophical and ethical positions on Therapeutic Recreation and your agency." (p. 5).

Professionals developing agency standards must also become aware of the weaknesses in the regulatory standards that are available. The most significant is that standards are made to apply to such a wide variety of health care facilities; thus, they tend to be too broad. In order for them to be more useful to the QA program, professionals must be able to make them more specific.

There are several reasons for developing specific agency standards. First, they can be written at a specific level geared toward therapeutic recreation service. Second, they can be written in a unique fashion, thus complementing your setting. Lastly, because agency standards are specifically

31

designed, there is greater control by department staff over the final evaluation. As an example, the JCAH standards are developed mainly by physicians and nurses with input from a variety of other activity services personnel. While recreation therapists and NTRS have input, they do not have control.

The Veterans Administration (VA) began developing agency standards in 1976 to provide their external surveyors with a more uniform approach for their audits. It was hoped that these standards would better measure the quality of care, provide problem identification, and permit more reliable analysis and comparisons of programs. Additionally, it was intended that these standards would provide a tool that could be used at any time at a medical center as a monitor of quality services. A basic seven-step process was used to develop recreation service standards:

1. The director, or representative, of the recreation service meets with agency experts to learn about the overall program.
2. The proposed draft is put together by subject-matter experts.
3. The proposed draft is sent to every medical center for comments and changes.
4. A second draft is completed by the original subject-matter experts.
5. Standards are field-tested and subject matter experts meet with agency standards experts.
6. The final draft is approved and instituted.
7. Standards are reviewed and changed annually to reflect changes in the profession and the agency.

The first set of standards includes eleven separate criteria with indicators and explanations for external auditors. These standards reflect the uniqueness of the agency, specific concerns of recreation services, and the state of the art as it is practiced at that time. The criteria are currently reviewed under the following headings:

1. Written policies and procedures,
2. Availability of sufficient resources,
3. Provision of comprehensive services,
4. Documentation of treatment,
5. Provision of innovative programs to meet assessed patient needs,
6. Quality Assurance programs,
7. Staff development programs,
8. Representation on medical center committees,
9. Effective leadership within the recreation service,
10. Documented clinical training programs,
11. Use of community resources.

Under each criteria are between three and ten indicators describing how they will be met, along with explanations to help guide the auditor (Johnson et al, 1984, pp. 59–61). This also allows for more control and input by professionals in the audit process. As an example, the aforementioned regulatory agencies (JCAH, CARF, etc.) have all required written policies and procedures; however, they have not proceeded beyond this point. In the VA agency standards, written policies and procedures provide the following:

1. Organizational alignment,
2. A mission statement that is consistent with Agency Mission,
3. Long- and short-range goals,
4. A description of treatment philosophy,
5. Policies that include at least the following:
   a. Assessment of Patient Needs,
   b. Guides for Program Planning,
   c. Patient Referral Procedures,
   d. Treatment Implementation Practices,
   e. Staff Development,
   f. Requirements for Patient Record Documentation,
   g. Clinical Privileges,
   h. Quality Assurance,
   i. Staff Meetings,
   j. Infection Control,
   k. Patient Incident Reporting,
   l. Off-station Field Trips,
   m. Disaster and Fire Preparedness,
   n. Property Control,
   o. Guidelines for Volunteers.

The above provides more specific guidelines in developing policies and procedures than do the agency standards of the regulatory agencies. The above approach also allows for individual agency flexibility in that it mentions policy areas but not specific policy content.

Conclusion. In summary, the therapeutic recreation professional must be aware of the regulatory agency's standards affecting his/her provision of services. He/she must also be aware of professional (NTRS) standards and keep abreast of these standards and revisions since they are ever-changing. As shown, one of the ways to make standards more meaningful is to write agency-specific standards. In developing these, professionals should remember the seven-step process. Once agency standards are developed, they must also be reviewed as regulatory and professional standards change.

The only constant in providing a quality assurance program is change. This is a necessity in order to provide state-of-the-art services that reflect professional and regulatory guidelines.

REFERENCES

Berryman, D. (1971). *Recommended Standards with Evaluative Criteria for Recreation Services in Residential Institutions.* New York, NY: New York University School of Education.

Commission on Accreditation of Rehabilitation Facilities (1986). *Standards Manual for Organizations Serving People with Disabilities.* Tucson, AZ.

Commission on Accreditation of Rehabilitation Facilities (1986). *The CARF Story.* Tucson, AZ.

Federal Register, Subpart J, Forty-Second Code (1976). Conditions of participation: Hospitals. Washington, DC: United States Government Printing Office.

Johnson, D., Donovan, G., Bellah, J., and Waterman, F. (1984). "Comprehensive Quality Assurance." In G. Hitzhusen (Ed.), *Expanding Horizons in Therapeutic Recreation XI* (pp. 56–65). University of Missouri.

Joint Commission on Accreditation of Hospitals (1986). *Ambulatory Health Care Standards Manual.* Chicago, IL.

Joint Commission on Accreditation of Hospitals (1986). *Long Term Care Manual.* Chicago, IL.

Joint Commission on Accreditation of Hospitals (1985). *Consolidated Standards Manual.* Chicago, IL.

Joint Commission on Accreditation of Hospitals (1985). *Consolidated Standards Manual for Child, Adolescent, and Adult Psychiatry, Alcoholism and Drug Abuse Facilities; and Facilities Serving MR/DD.* Chicago, IL.

Joint Commission on Accreditation of Hospitals (1983). *Hospice Standards Manual.* Chicago, IL.

Joint Commission on Accreditation of Hospitals (1980). *Accreditation Manual for Hospitals.* Chicago, IL.

LaBrenz, M. (Project ed.) (1985). *An Introduction to JCAH: Its Survey and Accreditation Process, Standards, and Services.* Chicago, IL: Joint Commission on Accreditation of Hospitals.

National Therapeutic Recreation Society (1980). *Guidelines for Administration of Therapeutic Recreation Service in Clinical and Residential Facilities.* Alexandria, VA: National Recreation and Park Association.

National Therapeutic Recreation Society (1980). *Standards of Practice for Therapeutic Recreation Service.* Alexandria, VA: National Recreation and Park Association.

Waterman, F. (1986). *One-Minute TR Manager.* Unpublished manuscript.

Waterman, F., Johnson, D., and Cantrell, J. (1981). "Criteria-based Quality Assurance in Multi-facility Organizations." In N. Navar and J. Dunn (Eds.), *Quality Assurance Concerns for Therapeutic Recreation* (pp. 117–181). University of Illinois.

IV. MEDICAL PEER REVIEW, THE GOVERNMENT, AND THE PRACTITIONER: PARTNERS IN QUALITY OF CARE

JAMES J. TICEHURST

With the advent of Medicare and Medicaid in 1965, the federal government established utilization review programs to ensure that health-care services it provided for were appropriate, efficiently provided, and of acceptable quality. Responsibility for utilization review in hospitals was vested in locally based Utilization Review Committees, either organized within the hospital by a substantial number of practitioners (physicians), or monitored by Department of Health, Education and Welfare-approved groups, which again included a substantial number of physicians. This basic theme formed the structure for the procedure of practitioners reviewing practitioners and medical services ordered or furnished by other practitioners. Such a concept, established for this prime purpose, has been the instrument by which the peer review system has functioned since its inception. In November, 1972, in an attempt to alleviate the inadequacies of the existing hospital utilization review program, Congress created the Professional Standards Review Organization (PSRO). Their intent was to improve the previous utilization review programs.

Since the PSRO Law was passed in 1972, many amendments to this legislation have been passed in a continuing effort to improve the program. These efforts resulted in a conglomeration of requirements which made the administration and evaluation of the PSRO program difficult, if not impossible. The program was subjected to, and continues to be subjected to, numerous evaluations which are often inconclusive or contradictory. These results have pointed out further shortcomings of the PSRO legislation; consistent and explicit performance criteria are necessary for the evaluation of the effectiveness of the program.

These recurring problems and the perceived need by Congress to maintain a system of accountability have led to the repeal of the PSRO program and the creation of peer-review organizations (PROs) in the formulation of the Tax Equity and Fiscal Responsibility Act (TEFRA) of 1982. Their actions are precipitated by the belief that the medical review system, while essential, needed a major restructuring. The PRO law retains the positive attributes of the PSRO program, eliminates the negative components and incorporates changes deemed necessary by previous experience.

The Peer Review Improvement Act of 1982 shows that the Congress believes that the concept of peer review is valid and that medical practitioners are capable and willing to work to assure the efficient and effective provision of health-care services that are of acceptable quality. In 1983, amendments to the Social Security laws changed the Medicare reimbursement basis for hospitals from a cost-based system to a prospective payment system (PPS) based on diagnosis-related groups, more commonly known as DRGs. Even in light of all the changes and legislative amendments, PROs continue to assume the responsibility for ensuring that the system is not abused and that the quality of care provided is not compromised. The required review activities and objectives of the PROs are designed to allow the accomplishment of these responsibilities.

As PROs, PSROs have had to modify many of the review functions which they formerly performed. Of major importance is perhaps the restrictions on the use of physicians in the review process. Specifically stated, a physician affiliated with a hospital may not perform utilization review activities on Medicare cases at that hospital. The intent is to insure an objective review by the PRO physician. Secondly, utilization review activities on Medicare cases should, whenever possible, be performed by physician specialists in the area under review. Again, the intent is to insure that cases requiring special medical consideration are being afforded that specialty. Along with restrictions of this type, PROs identify those areas of major concern within their own environment. Such consideration is given to issues of admission objectives, quality objectives of special concern, and local or statewide concentrations.

What, Then, Does a Typical PRO Resemble? The PSRO law was legislated and enacted on October 30, 1972, setting into motion a system to review and monitor medical care provided under Medicare and Medicaid. From 1972 to

1984, PSROs operated under grants funded by the Health Care Financing Administration, a division of the US Department of Health and Human Services. For the purpose of describing a relatively standard PSRO, the Vermont Professional Standards Review Organization, Inc., an organization currently in operation within the State of Vermont, will be used.

Although the Federal PSRO law took effect in 1972, planning and legislation for the Vermont PSRO was only accomplished between 1974 and 1976, with an official PSRO designation in 1976 and concurrent funding through the federal grants program.

Originally founded as a physician-based organization, Vermont PSRO membership consists of over six hundred licensed physicians currently practicing medicine within the boundaries of the state. Guiding the organization's operations is a twenty-eight member Board of Directors, fifteen of whom are physicians and thirteen non-physicians, most of whom are closely aligned with health care or consumer issues. Under the PSRO system, Vermont PSRO functions under contracts for Medicare and Medicaid reviews. Staffing currently consists of an administrative office, located in South Burlington, Vermont, and a field staff of review coordinators located in each of Vermont's sixteen acute-care hospitals, plus both psychiatric and specialty hospitals. In conjunction with a regulated random-sample review process of Medicare and Medicaid patients, VT PSRO administers a pre-admission program for evaluation and certification of specific surgical procedures for inpatient hospitalization.

From the period 1976 to 1981, VT PSRO performed functional medical review for both long-term care and acute care in all hospitals and nursing homes within the state. From 1981 to 1984, the organization performed review functions in only the acute care and specialty hospitals under the PSRO system. In order to be eligible to serve as a VT PSRO review physician, a physician must be a licensed, practicing physician in the State of Vermont, be approved by VT PSRO, and attend a review physicians training session(s), required by VT PSRO. Once a physician has fulfilled all of the above requirements, he/she is considered to be an approved review physician.

VT PSRO and the Quality of Care. Congress has charged peer-review organizations (PROs) with the duties and functions to assure that the quality of care provided to Medicare recipients meets "professionally recognized standards" of care as defined by HCFA in part B of Title XIX of the Social Security Act. Such duties and functions include the implementation and operation of a review system to eliminate unreasonable, unnecessary and inappropriate care provided to Medicare beneficiaries and to assure the quality of services for which payment may be made. The PRO approach, designed to outline their responsibilities to assure that quality of care is being afforded to the patient, relies on several factors, most notably the physician reviewers' sense of what constitutes professionally recognized standards. Systematically, the PRO will pursue the identification of issues by the professionals reviewing cases, discussion with attending physician(s) for educational interaction, interaction with hospital Peer Review Committees, if a more formal educational program is needed, and, finally, action steps by the PRO whenever necessary. Thus, the peer-review organization will implement interventions whenever a quality issue is identified, to include denial of payment, if appropriate, educational interventions, intensified review, and possible sanctions, which may include physician(s) and/or hospital(s).

Briefly, the components outlined by the VT PSRO in the step-by-step quality process are:

1. The identification of questions that address quality issues as raised by VT PSRO review physicians
2. The evaluation of the quality issue (using severity indices)
3. The intervention of time frames and sequencing
4. Implementation of action steps, when appropriate, including educational interactions with hospitals and/or physicians
5. Data-system record-keeping

Generic-quality screens and generic discharge screens, effective November, 1986, are applied to all medical records reviewed for any reason by the VT PSRO. Should a case fail one or more of the screens, it is identified as a possible quality issue and automatically referred to a review physician for further review and evaluation. The purpose of the evaluation is to determine the severity of the quality-of-care issue. Once a quality issue has been raised, a dialogue is established between the VT PSRO Review Physician and the attending physician(s) and proceeds carefully from one step to the next, following the precise outline established by the review organization. Some case will require very little follow-up after the initial discussions between the review physician and attending physician, while in other cases the issue may require whatever steps are necessary to resolve the issue, and may go as far as a sanction action. In all cases where a quality-of-care issue has been raised, the PSRO must retain, for record-keeping purposes, important information on the case as a basis for data collection. This information must include the issue raised, the review physician's concerns and questions, the practitioner's response, the hospital response, if necessary, the medical director's evaluation, the evaluation by the PSRO Quality of Care Committee, the type of problem, the assigned severity index and the actions taken, and all correspondence relating to the case.

In all cases, the process is mandated by a rigid confidentiality policy strictly adhered to all PSRO's. This process is intended to point out any quality deficiencies in our system and so we may act on them accordingly. In this way the PSRO and the government can safely assure the patient that quality of care is being afforded to all in the prescribed manner.

Quality of Care and Therapeutic Recreation. There is perhaps no better time than now to discuss additional benefits to our health-care system. During the conference on the "Evaluation of Therapeutic Recreation through Quality Assurance," I mentally noted the dedication and the expressed concern from conference participants as they addressed a key question facing them, that is, "Where do we fit in?" It is not simply the exploration of the need for implementing effective quality assurance programs within the therapeutic recreation system, but more so the issue of how to implement effective therapeutic recreation programs within the quality of care program.

As we continue to acknowledge the need to develop and refine patient-care programs, we find new and expanded ways of assessing and measuring the outcomes of quality of care. Cooperatively within this assessment, we are approaching new ways of delivering additional services to strengthen that quality system. In a time of innovation, research and the development of rehabilitation services are becoming of greater importance. Therapeutic recreation, as near as one can tell, appears to be a function which may become of paramount importance in the quality system. However, it is also clear that many who deal directly in the monitoring and administration of the health system know little, if anything, about this kind of delivery service. It can also be stated with some degree of certainty, that unless therapeutic recreation professionals make their presence known, there is very little that will be accomplished in providing this service in the distant future.

As suggested in my presentation at the conference, the best way of making this happen is to contact your Health Care Financing Administration (HCFA) Regional Office or communicate with your state PRO. Their location can be found by contacting most hospitals within your state. If there is truly a desire to move forward with your goal of gaining status as a viable and necessary provider within the health-care system, then it is precisely the right time to move forward and make your presence felt. In this time of new ideas, therapeutic recreation may be one of the new ways of providing medical services, or at the very least quality services. Whether we are providers, monitors, or regulators, we are all players with the driving force to provide quality care to the patient while eliminating unnecessary costs or inappropriate care. In the time ahead, let us all move toward that common goal.

Quality of Care and the Future. There has never been a time in the history of the health-care system when so much emphasis has been placed on the quality of medical care, and rightfully so. It seems that all parties and participants within the system are collectively striving for more accountability when quality is the issue. In the passing months, there has been extensive concentration on and discussion about the growing concern for quality of care. There has been much federal rhetoric about the need to strengthen the regulations designed to monitor quality of care in the health system, generating numerous legislative drafts of proposed amendments to laws affecting health-care recipients. Those of notable mention are the Heinz-Stark Draft Comprehensive Medical Quality Assurance Act and the Durenburger Subcommittee hearings on health-care issues. However, no matter what the issue, the major focal point for all discussion centers on the quality of care afforded to the patient. As for the PROs, the spillover is seen in the current negotiations for contract renewals, with the emphasis on quality issues within the expanded scope of work for the next contract periods. Such expansion would:

1. provide for more depth in the review of quality of care in hospitals
2. require PROs to do quality assurance beyond the hospital door
3. require PROs to distribute information on quality-assurance activities and findings.

These potential requirements, as well as others, have surfaced as a byproduct of quality concerns. The necessity to concentrate on these issues is justified; however, one must not lose sight of the overall goal. For those who provide, for those who pay, for those who monitor and for those who legislate, the task is never-ending. By attempting to provide the best health-care system on earth at the lowest possible cost with the greatest benefit to those who use it— and still abide by the regulations that control it—is something to think about. As strange as it all seems, it appears to be working.

V. THERAPEUTIC RECREATION'S WRITTEN PLAN OF OPERATION: THE STEP *BEFORE* QUALITY ASSURANCE

NANCY NAVAR

In a general sense, all therapeutic recreation practitioners certainly believe in the concept of quality assurance in the provision of therapeutic recreation services. Specifically, accreditation organizations such as the Joint Commission on Accreditation of Hospitals (JCAH) outline processes and structures for documenting quality assurance in clinical settings. Many therapeutic recreation practitioners are presently trying to operationalize their general belief in quality services while simultaneously attempting to comply with accreditation standards provided by JCAH. Many times this task seems enormous.

Occasionally even the best-intentioned staff becomes frustrated when attempting to explain or develop their department's quality-assurance plan and procedures. An exemplary quality-assurance plan of two years ago may even be outdated. In this instance, updating may consist of the relatively simple task of converting from a *problem-oriented* quality-assurance procedure to the newer *monitoring* quality-assurance system. In another instance, therapeutic recreation staff may be attempting to design a quality-assurance procedure before they have thoroughly examined their therapeutic recreation program and its functioning within the agency. This particular staff will need to back up a bit and complete some prerequisite professional "homework" before they have sufficient information to complete a usable departmental quality-assurance plan. This paper focuses on the latter example cited above and attempts to explain how clinical therapeutic recreation departments can prepare to develop a usable quality-assurance plan.

Professional Updating. Before presenting the content of a written plan of operation, it is important to look briefly at the reason for documentation in general: to improve the quality of client services. Riley's presentation attempted to define/describe quality in a broad sense while Huston's presentation specifically addresses JCAH's new quality-assurance process. Here we'll briefly look at the resources that are available to help therapeutic recreation practitioners address/define/explain quality therapeutic-recreation services.

One resource available to assist in the determination of a quality therapeutic-recreation program is *client input*. However, most professions recognize that client input alone is insufficient to determine either the quality or the appropriateness of a professional service. Another resource that is useful in defining quality is the identification of *client needs*. Different professionals have different opinions about these, yet an opinion is much less valid than a formal assessment. In general, we can say that if a therapeutic-recreation program successfully addresses assessed client needs, it has aspects of being a quality program. But what if the assessment is too narrow in scope or addresses inappropriate content? An assessment that only measures recreation activity interests could hardly be considered a state-of-the-art clinical therapeutic-recreation assessment.

No matter how quality therapeutic-recreation services are defined, the accuracy of that description depends on the degree that therapeutic recreation's professional body of knowledge is being utilized; that is, is quality being defined using state-of-the-art professional information, or is quality being defined based on department tradition and uninformed staff opinion? Therapeutic recreation professionals have an obligation to stay current with their professional body of knowledge. They have an obligation to use the available professional documents to help define quality therapeutic-recreation programs.

Current advanced-level therapeutic-recreation textbooks provide up-to-date information that may not have been available just a few years earlier.[1] Professional organizations' newsletters frequently provide information that can relate to the identification of quality therapeutic-recreation services.[2] Professional journals and specialty publications are additional resources used by all human service professions.[3] The JCAH expects that each professional keeps up to date in his or her own professional area of expertise. (The Joint Commission emphasizes this so much that recent standards require that quality-assurance results be tied directly to staff reappointment and staff privileges.) Unless a therapeutic recreation practitioner is professionally up to date, any attempt at defining quality will be limited and less than ideal.

Each therapeutic recreation practitioner should also familiarize him- or herself with one additional resource: the accreditation manual used by the agency. Receiving a xeroxed copy of one or two pages of standards that directly address therapeutic recreation is not sufficient. There are standards throughout the entire manual that affect therapeutic-recreation services.

After a professional assumes responsibility for keeping current within his or her own profession, the reading and interpretation of accreditation standards manuals has some professional reference point. While JCAH standards manuals at times appear vague, that generality is intentional. More and more, JCAH is expecting that each discipline will interpret the standards from their own professional frame of reference. For example, the Joint Commission will not define quality therapeutic-recreation services because it expects that therapeutic-recreation practitioners will read and interpret JCAH structure and process standards and add to them current state-of-the-art therapeutic-recreation content. Very bluntly, any profession that fails to define quality services is in great jeopardy.

Each JCAH accreditation manual (Hospital, Consolidated, Long Term Care, etc.) has identical quality-assurance standards. These standards no longer focus on problems. Instead, each *department* must determine the most important aspects of patient care and regularly monitor these. The therapeutic-recreation practitioner assumes the responsibility for defining and monitoring quality care from a therapeutic-recreation perspective.

In summary, the most important resources available for defining quality therapeutic-recreation services are the therapeutic-recreation literature that is available. In addition to current text and specialty books, most of this literature is available through the National Therapeutic Recreation Society and the American Therapeutic Recreation Association. A second critical resource is the accreditation manual. Each JCAH standards manual provides similar quality-assurance requirements, yet therapeutic-recreation departments must define quality services for their own department based on professional expertise.

The quality-assurance process, as defined by JCAH, includes the following steps. First, the Joint Commission expects that the staff who are planning the quality-assurance process are competent to do so; that is, the staff are professionally educated, have the proper credentials, and are currently competent in their particular discipline. Assuming such competence, the actual first step in the quality-assurance process is the determination of the most important aspects of client care. Although many functions and tasks performed by therapeutic recreation staff can be considered important, each department should narrow the chief aspects of patient care to possibly four to seven items. For example, in therapeutic-recreation services, client assessment, involvement in the treatment plan, provision of a comprehensive program (therapy, leisure education, and recreation participation), and accurate progress notes may be one agency's summary of the four most important aspects of client care.

The second major step in JCAH's suggested quality-assurance process is the determination of objective criteria that will directly represent each of the important aspects of client care. Once again, this criteria should be based on current professional knowledge and clinical experience. Huston's article expands on this step and provides several examples of indicators and criteria related to the important aspects of client care.

The third major step in JCAH's suggested quality-assurance process is the determination of the monitoring methods. Basically, therapeutic-recreation specialists determine how they will monitor or keep track of the important aspects of client care since much documentation that is presently being collected by staff seems to be busy work. This documentation really doesn't tell the staff very much, and the date often gets filed without being used. Thus a monitoring step of the quality-assurance process enables each department to decide which documentation really is important and useful, helping professionals to streamline the total record collecting process. In many ways, departments now have more control over what information is collected, how it is collected, and how the information is used. If during this monitoring process a client-care problem arises, the department has several choices of what to do next. The problem issue can be justified, the problem can be corrected, or the problem can be further studied and then corrected. The older problem-focused approach to quality assurance still is quite useful when there is actually a client-care problem. In other words, the problem-solving methods of quality assurance are still needed; what's different now is that quality assurance includes much more than problem-solving.

The fourth major aspect of JCAH's suggested process for quality assurance is the evaluation of the entire monitoring process. Therapeutic recreation specialists must make some objective judgments on whether the important aspects of client care are being implemented at acceptable levels; they must make some judgments about the findings and conclusions of the monitoring and problem-solving activities that the department has done; they must integrate their departmental quality-assurance monitoring into the total agency quality-assurance program.

This quality-assurance process and the procedures involved in the process are both made easier when therapeutic recreation staff understand the total functioning of their department; that is, how does the therapeutic recreation department fit into the entire agency? What procedures are done for client care and what procedures are done solely because they are required by administration? What documentation is needed and what documentation is a duplication of effort and could be eliminated? To answer these and other prospective questions, the therapeutic recreation staff must comprehensively take a look at each aspect of their department functioning. One way of clarifying a department's role within an agency is to develop a departmental therapeutic-recreation written plan of operation. This written plan provides a framework from which a therapeutic-recreation department is very accountable and integrated within the agency. In many ways, the written plan of operation is actually prerequisite to the quality-assurance plan. In some instances, staff may be formulating both simultaneously. Either way, the written plan is an important ingredient in departmental efficiency.

The Written Plan. Although many therapeutic-recreation departments do have policy and procedure manuals that document both general and specific items, few of these manuals would actually qualify as comprehensive departmental written plans. Certainly, a policy and procedure manual would be included in a department's written plan; yet a plan of operation is much more comprehensive than a policy and procedure manual, much broader in scope and more detailed. This written plan must be more descriptive of the actual clinical functioning of the department within the overall agency and include such items as communications, referrals, time lines, and other program-and client-management procedures that occur in a clinical setting.

Two major types of clinical written plans of operation are of concern to therapeutic-recreation practitioners: first, the overall agency (hospital, rehabilitation center, etc.) should have a written plan of operation that includes therapeutic recreation; second, the therapeutic-recreation department (activity therapy, recreation therapy, etc.) needs to have a written plan of operation for department or unit functioning.

The Agency-written Plan of Operation. Accreditation surveyors typically review an agency's written plan of operation quite thoroughly. If therapeutic recreation is not adequately included in this plan, accreditation surveyors will probably not look upon therapeutic recreation as a major agency service. The responsibility for including therapeutic recreation in an agency's written plan of operation belongs to the therapeutic-recreation administrator. Each of these administrators should become familiar with the agency's written plan of operation, both content and format, and provide suggestions on how therapeutic recreation may be addressed in all relevant sections of the plan. Although agency plans will vary in both content and format, the following functions are often included.

1. *Patient management functions.* Patient management includes procedures such as intake, client assessment, treatment plans, progress notes, treatment plan reviews ("staffings"), discharge summaries and aftercare. Although it is generally desirable for therapeutic recreation to be mentioned

in several sections of the agency's written plan, two types of statements are particularly crucial during an era of service cutbacks and tight budgets. These critical statements concern therapeutic recreation's involvement in client *assessment* and *treatment plans.* Sample statements that might be included in the agency's plan are as follows.

"Therapeutic recreation services are an integral part of the treatment process." A statement such as this is documented testimony that therapeutic recreation belongs in the treatment plan, that therapeutic recreation is a bona fide treatment modality—not just a support service—and that therapeutic recreation has a definitive role within the agency. Another statement that can be quite powerful for assuring the future existence and functioning of therapeutic recreation is: "The recreation/leisure assessment is conducted by a Certified Therapeutic Recreation Specialist." Such a statement can be a form of insurance. Since accreditation standards do not specify who will conduct the recreation/leisure assessment, there is no guarantee that it will be conducted by a therapeutic-recreation professional unless the agency makes such a statement/commitment. Although such statements concerning therapeutic recreation's involvement in treatment plans and client assessments will not necessarily ensure therapeutic recreation's future, the absence of such statements does endanger the future existence of some therapeutic-recreation departments. Thus it is quite important that such statements be documented in the agency's written plan of operation in addition to therapeutic recreation's departmental written plan.

2. *Program-management functions.* Program-management functions should also be addressed in the agency's written plan of operation. Program-management functions include quality-assurance activities, patient-care monitoring, utilization reviews, staff growth and development activities, research activities and patient rights.

Very frequently, agencies do not include detailed descriptions of each department's involvement in these activities in the overall agency written plan. Yet the more integrated therapeutic-recreation departments frequently have regular or periodic involvement in many of these program-management functions. Whenever possible, the therapeutic-recreation administrator should attempt to document therapeutic recreation's involvement in these program-management activities in the overall agency written plan.

The Therapeutic Recreation Written Plan of Operation. A self-regulating, professional therapeutic-recreation department should have a comprehensive department-level written plan of operation. As accreditation standards become less and less prescriptive, it becomes more important for each discipline to accurately describe its purpose and function within the overall agency. Frequently, it is this departmental document that facilitates entry into the overall agency written plan of operation. In the near future, it will be this departmental level document, in conjunction with the agency written plan, that will describe that profession's degree of accountability and contribution to quality client care.

The following questions and comments are presented as guidelines for developing a therapeutic-recreation written plan of operation. A document to be read thoroughly before answering these questions is the National Therapeutic Recreation Society's *Standards of Practice for Therapeutic Recreation Service*.

1. What is the philosophy of therapeutic recreation at your specific agency? NTRS and/or ATRA philosophical statements can serve as a foundation for a department's philosophy, yet each agency will have to specifically define the philosophy of that agency's therapeutic-recreation service.

2. What are the goals of the comprehensive therapeutic-recreation program in a specific agency? Global, unmeasurable goals are no longer acceptable. Each program's goals should directly relate to an implemented program component.

3. What are the components of the comprehensive therapeutic-recreation service? Many therapeutic-recreation departments are using therapy, leisure education, and recreation participation. Other components are equally acceptable, i.e., community resources, leisure awareness and skill development of social activities, solitary activities and communication skills, etc.). The appropriateness of these components varies by agency type and predominant client characteristics.

    Components should be broad enough in scope to permit specific program changes to occur without rewriting program components. For example, a department that chooses bowling, aquatics, and table games does not allow for much program change. This department is really encouraging additional unnecessary documentation since the written plan of operation must be updated to correspond to actual program offerings.

    Goals should be specified for each program component. When the therapeutic-recreation department's written plan includes specific component goals and corresponding behavioral objectives, treatment plans and charting are often simplified. If the written plan of operation contains a wide range of possible client objectives, then the documenting of objectives in the client's chart becomes less time-consuming.

4. How do clients become involved in each program component? Some agencies may use a physician referral process while others may use voluntary participation by clients. The method of involving clients can vary for each program component. The written plan of operation simply spec-

ifies which methods are used to involve clients in the therapeutic-recreation services.

5. What specific programs are provided by the therapeutic-recreation department? Again, many therapeutic-recreation staff can lessen their documentation requirements by explaining broader program concepts behind specific activities. Any given therapeutic-recreation department can offer hundreds of activities. It is an overwhelming and unnecessary task to attempt to document all the details of every activity offering. Yet it is a responsible and wise move to document, in the written plan of operation, the specific purposes and procedures for each program offering.

   For example, a specific program offering might be "leisure awareness." This could include values-clarification activities and leisure decision-making and planning sessions. A "social skills" program might include assertiveness, effective-listening, or telephone-etiquette activities. A written plan of operation would explain each program offering and list possible activities that are used in the various programs.

6. How are specific programs and the comprehensive program evaluated? How often does this evaluation occur? Whether formal or informal evaluation procedures are used, they should be explained in the written plan of operation. A function as routine as a staff meeting can be one valid method of program evaluation if it is documented as such.

7. What type of client assessment is used? How is it used for program placement, referral, etc.)? When is it used? For what type of client on what functional level is it used? (Different types of clients may receive different types of assessments.) Who is qualified to perform therapeutic recreation client assessments? How are those qualifications documented and reviewed?

8. What policies, procedures or forms are utilized by the therapeutic recreation department?

9. How does therapeutic recreation interact with other professional services? For example, a therapeutic-recreation written plan might indicate that therapeutic recreation provides an interdisciplinary swim program with physical therapy. In this case, a short description of interdisciplinary functioning and methods of communication should also be documented. In addition, the physical therapy department's written plan of operation should indicate a similar interdisciplinary swim program with the therapeutic-recreation department.

10. What is the role of therapeutic recreation in relation to patient management functions? Included in the therapeutic-recreation written plan of operation are the procedures used when therapeutic recreation is involved in: client intake, client assessment, treatment plans, progress notes, treatment plan reviews, discharge summaries, and aftercare. A comprehensive strategy that some therapeutic-recreation administrators

50

use is the documentation of patient-management functions that do NOT involve therapeutic-recreation services. This ensures that the reader of the written plan of operation—i.e., administrator, surveyor, etc.— understand exactly which clinical functions involve therapeutic-recreation staff and which do not.

11. What is the role of therapeutic recreation in relation to program-management functions? As stated earlier, program-management functions include quality-assurance activities, patient-care monitoring, utilization reviews, staff growth and development activities, research activities, and patient rights. The therapeutic-recreation written plan of operation should indicate which of these functions involve therapeutic recreation staff and which do not. When therapeutic recreation participates in a particular program-management function, the details of that participation should be explained in the written plan.

The preceding questions can serve as guidelines for the content of a therapeutic-recreation written plan of operation. Formats for such written plans should be agency specific. When choosing a format and an organizational method for documenting and updating the information contained in the written plan, keep in mind that usability is quite important. No one wants to spend hours creating a document that collects dust and does not serve a functional purpose. Separate looseleaf notebooks are one method that seems to be widely used. A "master" notebook includes an outline of all available documented information. Then separate notebooks are organized for such categories as personnel information, program information, patient management, program management, and quality assurance. Each agency or department decides the most useful method for organizing the entire written plan.

Timelines and Reasonable Expectations. The task of documenting a comprehensive written plan of operation is a lengthy process. Therapeutic-recreation departments that did not have a written plan yesterday will not have one tomorrow since no therapeutic-recreation department can be expected to design a comprehensive, usable written plan of operation overnight. Therefore, the therapeutic-recreation administrator should first conceptualize the content and format of the written plan of operation. This "master plan" can then be included in the beginning of the written plan of operation. (Such a form of planning is also appropriate at the agency level.[4]) Included in the "master plan" or implementation plan should be a realistic timeline for the completion of the comprehensive written plan of operation.

The written plan can be viewed as an insurance policy. Regardless of whether external pressure is present, the "insured" therapeutic recreation department should start the process of documenting what they do, why they do it, how they do it, and how well it's working. Professional services should also initiate such efforts rather than waiting for administrative directives. When one waits for administrative directives, the resultant posture is typically reactive rather than proactive. Successful clinical functioning requires proactive staff who are able to function within their professional specialty while remaining fully aware of the larger agency environment. Without such a perspective, quality-assurance plans will lack relevance and depth. After a therapeutic-recreation department spends the weeks and months needed to comprehensively explain their operation, the identification of a quality-assurance plan will be a relatively less complicated task.

In summary, the first task of each professional is to make certain that he or she is professionally up-to-date by reading and utilizing the available professional resources such as NTRS Standards of Practice, etc.[5] The second step involves reviewing the accreditation standards manual that is being used by the overall agency. Professionals must interpret these standards from a therapeutic-recreation perspective, making certain that all of them throughout the entire manual are addressed. The third step is to take some time to think about the clinical activities that already involve therapeutic-recreation staff and programs. The fourth and most comprehensive step is to conceptualize the content for the therapeutic-recreation written plan of operation, beginning with the most familiar clinical activities. Professionals should start with what is understood and leave the major problems for later. (Many of these problems could eventually become part of the quality-assurance process.) During or after the formulation of a comprehensive written plan, they should determine the quality-assurance process that will be utilized by their therapeutic-recreation department.

Many therapeutic-recreation departments already have made progress in determining a useful quality assurance process. Some self-regulating professionals are taking the initiative and beginning to document a written plan of operation for therapeutic recreation. Still others are polishing and expanding old policy-and-procedure manuals and updating them to become written plans. Whatever degree of documentation exists in a particular therapeutic-recreation department, the documentation should be functional. Usefulness and efficiency of effort seem to be unspoken criteria in the quality-assurance process. Usefulness also seems to be a major key in translating therapeutic recreation's general concern for quality assurance into specific compliance with quality-assurance standards.

NOTES

[1]Two exceptional current textbooks are: Peterson, C.A. and S.L. Gunn (1984), *Therapeutic Recreation Program Design Principles and Procedures* (New Jersey: Prentice

Hall), and Reynolds, R.P. and G.S. O'Morrow, (1985), *Problems, Issues and Concepts in Therapeutic Recreation* (New Jersey: Prentice Hall).

²*American Therapeutic Recreation Association Newsletter*, c/o ATRA 2000 0 St. N.W., Washington, D.C. 20036, 202–457–0232, and *National Therapeutic Recreation Association Newsletter*, c/o NTRS 3101 Park Center Dr., Alexandria, VA 22302, 703–820–4940.

³The major professional journal in therapeutic recreation is *Therapeutic Recreation Journal*, c/o NTRS, 3101 Park Center Dr., Alexandria, VA 22302. A newer journal (formerly conference proceedings) is the *Journal of Expanding Horizons*, c/o Dept. of Recreation and Park Admin., 613 Clark Hall, University of Missouri, Columbia, MO 65211, 314–882–7086. First release date is late 1986. Specialty publications focus on a specific topic, a specific disability group or specific settings/services. A recent book that has relevance beyond long-term care settings is Carruthers, C., Sneegas, J.J., and C. Ashton-Shaeffer, (1986), *Therapeutic Recreation: Guidelines for Activity Services in Long Term Care*, Dept. of Leisure Studies, University of Illinois, 104 Huff Hall, 1206 S. Fourth St., Champaign, IL 61820 ($12.50 check payable to Univ. of Illinois).

⁴The Joint Commission has specific guidelines for "implementation monitoring" at the agency level.

⁵Documents that should be reviewed by each therapeutic recreation department include: *Standards of Practice for Therapeutic Recreation Service* (1980), *Guidelines for Administration of Therapeutic Recreation Service in Clinical and Residential Facilities* (1980), *Standards for Field Placement in Therapeutic Recreation* (1986). The preceding documents are available for a fee from the National Therapeutic Recreation Society, 3101 Park Center Dr., Alexandria, VA 22302. Additionally, each therapeutic recreation department should be familiar with the national credentialing program for therapeutic recreation. An explanation of the certification program and applications can be obtained from the National Council for Therapeutic Recreation Certification, P.O. Box 16126, Alexandria, VA 22302, 703–820–3993.

REFERENCES

Joint Commission on Accreditation of Hospitals (1985). *Accreditation Manual for Hospitals, Consolidated Standards Manual, Long Term Care Standards Manual.* Chicago, IL.

Joint Commission on Accreditation of Hospitals (1986). *Quality Assurance in Long Term Care.* Chicago, IL.

Navar, N. (1984). "Documentation in Therapeutic Recreation." In C.A. Peterson and S.L. Gunn, *Therapeutic Recreation Program Design: Principles and Procedures.* Englewood Cliffs, NJ: Prentice-Hall, Inc.

Navar, N. (1984). "Therapeutic Recreation Standards and a Written Plan of Operation." In G. Hitzhusen (Ed.), *Expanding Horizons in Therapeutic Recreation X*. Columbia, MO: University of Missouri.

Reynolds, R.P. and O'Morrow, G.S. (1985). *Problems, Issues and Concepts in Therapeutic Recreation*. Englewood Cliffs, NJ: Prentice-Hall, Inc.

VI. QUALITY ASSESSMENT: PRACTICAL APPROACHES IN THERAPEUTIC RECREATION

STEVEN WRIGHT

Quality assurance (QA) has emerged as the premier topic in the health-care industry. This is evidenced by the current wave of literature, conference-agenda, and agency-level discussions devoted to the theme of quality. In the late '70's, it was cost containment that took center stage as the industry wrestled with spiraling health-care costs. Today, the issue of quality care is of foremost interest to both provider and consumer. In fact, it is the cost issue that has helped spark an unprecedented interest in assuring that a minimum standard of quality care be provided to all patients regardless of the economic climate of health services.

Primary and ancillary services are inseparable elements of the health-care delivery system. Arguably, some of these services (e.g., surgery) are more immediate to a patient's health status and well-being than others. However, they all have an impact on the quality of patient care, so each should be systematically monitored and evaluated to assure acceptable standards of quality care. All health-care professions are faced with both the challenge and the responsibility to develop effective measures of the quality and appropriateness of their professional behavior and practice.

In respect to the therapeutic-recreation (TR) field, the profession needs to conceptualize, develop, and implement QA systems which reflect state-of-the-art TR practice. This requires a thorough understanding of the TR process and familiarity with quality assessment approaches and methods. Quality assessment is the operational arm of quality assurance; it is the fundamental process by which the quality of patient-care services is measured.

The specific objective of this paper is to discuss the quality-assessment process from organizational structure to application in the TR setting. It will not address the broader conceptual themes of quality and quality assurance, for these subjects are thoroughly covered elsewhere. Instead, this paper will focus on how to operationalize the varied elements of quality assessment and develop assessment activities appropriate for your setting.

Quality Assessment. Contrary to the fears of many administrators, planning, implementing, and evaluating quality-assessment activities within a well-defined TR program does not require the design and implementation of a totally new evaluation system. Many of the tools necessary for conducting quality assessment are readily available within the existing administrative framework of most therapeutic-recreation departments. For example, program evaluation, productivity analysis, performance appraising, and other administrative activities closely parallel quality-assessment activities. However, quality assessment is a distinct organizational function that should be designated as the primary focus of the department with other administrative functions revolving around this core activity. This would demonstrate the commitment of the TR department to providing quality patient-care services. (See Figure 6.1.)

Quality assessment is a systematic process of collecting targeted data, analyzing and comparing the data against pre-determined standards, taking appropriate action if necessitated, and optimally managing the entire quality review operation. Based on systems methodology, a specific functional model can be created to illustrate the "interrelated" steps of the quality-assessment process. (See Figure 6.2.) Primary organizational elements entail data-gathering (system inputs), the analysis of information system transformation), and the use of study results (system outputs).

Quality Assessment Model.

A. *Information Gathering.* Knowing where relevant information exists is essential to quality-of-care measurement. Information can be obtained retrospectively, concurrently, and/or prospectively from both existing patient-care data sources and/or obtained from newly generated sources of data. Some data sources include:

1. Patient Records—traditionally the richest source of patient-care data frequently used in conducting quality assessment. Patient documentation is evidence of the type and extent of the patient-care process.

Figure 6.1 Quality Assessment Organization

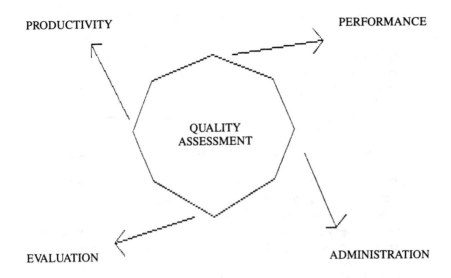

PRODUCTIVITY   PERFORMANCE

QUALITY
ASSESSMENT

EVALUATION   ADMINISTRATION

Figure 6.2 QA Organizational Functions

INFORMATION GATHERING	INFORMATION ANALYSIS	INFORMATION USE	OVERSIGHT SUPERVISION
1. Inputs	1. Practice Patterns	1. Action	1. Optimal and
2. Process	2. Resource Use	2. Problem Focused	Continuous
3. Outcome	3. General Trends	Review	Monitoring

2. Recreation Management System—existing information collected by the department. Examples include the number and types of services and programs conducted, attendance records, progress notes, and other data-collection sources.

3. Institutional Data Systems—agency management's wealth of data that is usually under-utilized by the therapeutic-recreation department. Results of utilization reviews and readmission data are two examples of readily available information that should be accessed for quality-assessment activities.

57

4. Sentinel Events—major events recorded as they happen within the quality-assurance system, e.g., incident reports. These may include the frequency of negative events—e.g., injury—late referrals, and missing documentation.

5. Staff Meetings—concerns and issues raised by staff. These are extremely important sources of data that may not be found in any of the above sources or detected by any other quality assessment mechanism.

With several mechanisms available for collecting quality-assessment data, choosing the best approach depends on the type of evaluation, requisite data, and time-and-money constraints. Data-collection mechanisms include:

1. Record Review—The classic "medical audit" uses documented information in the patient's medical charts to assess the practice patterns of the therapeutic-recreation practitioner.
2. Utilization Review—Here the focus is on the consumption of TR department resources with respect to time, personnel patterns, facility use, and equipment use.
3. Direct Observation—In the TR profession, observing practitioners may produce information not obtainable from documented sources. The process can entail a formal peer-review program or the day-to-day observation of a supervisor.
4. Client Surveys and Interviews—direct survey or interview of patients and patients' families with respect to the "consumer's perspective" (i.e., patient satisfaction) is very important to assessing the quality of the TR service.
5. Research—Departments can develop valid performance standards and establish criteria by which compliance can be measured through in-house-sponsored research activities. Studies could produce data particularly useful in refining assessment strategies and improving the overall QA program.

B. *Information Analysis.* After gathering desired information, the next step is to examine the data and give specific attention to variations in practice patterns, resource use, and general trends. The objective of the analysis is to identify any differences between actual practices and pre-established "norms." If the analysis raises a "flag," an assessment of the causes and impacts should be initiated on a case-by-case basis. Recommendations for future action to resolve the situation should also be clearly documented.

C. *Information Use.* Once a problem or potential problem has been identified through information analysis, timely and appropriate action must be taken to correct the situation. The area of concern might require a "problem-focused study" to examine the specific issue in greater detail, thus producing specific recommendations for change. This includes the key phase of problem resolution and ensuring that potential adverse patient impacts are minimized in the future. Action strategies designed to reduce the occurrence of further problems might be in the area of continuing education, certification, and/or administrative change.

D. *System Supervision.* The above-mentioned organizational structure provides a clear outline of the major functions of quality assessment. The ideal quality-assurance program is a planned and systematic process of monitoring and evaluating the major aspects of patient care through quality-assessment activities. The above-mentioned components of quality assessment must be supervised with unyielding attention to objectivity, reliability, responsiveness, comprehensiveness, and effectiveness. This process must be optimally managed to reflect state-of-the-art methods and approaches to measuring the quality of patient care services in therapeutic recreation.

Matrix-of-quality Decisions. The quality of direct patient care provided by therapeutic recreators is dependent upon many factors: professional training; years of experience; personal motivation and commitment; setting; etc. These factors are basic professional characteristics which have an immediate impact on the daily provision of service. Thus an important QA question is, how do these factors come together so that they collectively influence the quality of professional involvement in the TR treatment process?

Throughout the TR treatment routine, key decisions are made by the practitioner which have an impact on the quality of both the process itself and the outcome of care. These decisions are made at major stages of the TR procedure: assessment, treatment planning, treatment monitoring, discharge planning, and follow-up. Through closer examination of the treatment process, these quality relevant "decision points" can be identified according to applicable activities. For example, Figure 6.3 illustrates the common activities and central questions the practitioner must address during the assessment phase. These questions include: 1) What type of treatment does the patient need? 2) What specific services should the patient receive? 3) What staff member should provide the basic services? 4) Who should manage the overall treatment plan? The decision-making process requires the practitioner to draw upon "professional expertise" and make responsible choices based on acceptable practice patterns. These decisions, to a greater or lesser extent, directly affect the quality of both the process of providing care and the outcome of the intervention.

These questions or decision points represent critical areas of evaluation with respect to quality assessment. Clear identification of the decision points in a TR program is an important step that can help sharpen a QA program

Figure 6.3 Assessment Activities and Decisions

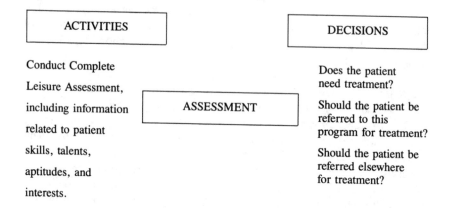

focus. Concentrating on information useful to improving the effectiveness of future decisions can ultimately improve the quality of care rendered.

Indicators, Criteria, and Standards. Decision points provide a good reference for further defining quality-assessment activities within a TR program. As the profession builds on its professional knowledge base, it must also refine its operational approaches to measuring the quality of therapeutic intervention. This can only be accomplished by targeting important indicators, formulating measurement criteria, and specifying standards of acceptable practice. To assure consistency and clarity, the following terms are defined for the remaining discussion (Donabedian, 1982).

Major aspect of care: Represents the "critical elements" of a service.

Indicator: Specifies the patient-care activities, events, occurrences, and outcomes that are to be monitored and evaluated.

Criteria: Can be any aspect of structure, process, or outcome that has a bearing on the overall quality of care. These are explicit, objective, generally accepted measures of appropriateness and quality.

Standard: Precise, quantitative specification of a criterion that constitutes quality of a given degree.

The TR treatment model provides a framework for viewing the most important aspects of TR services and care. It is within this model that the profession must distinguish the patient-care activities or indicators that should be monitored. Indicators are usually framed in terms of appropriateness, adequacy, timeliness, intensity, compliance, etc. of some aspect of care.

Given identified indicators, criteria, and standards should then be established to assess the level of quality. Criteria and standards are often woven together in one statement so that the criteria becomes both a measurement approach as well as explicit standards of acceptable practice. However, criteria and standards may also become vague and ambiguous when combined. Therefore it is more appropriate to formulate them independently of each other and give particular attention to valid measurement design and professionally acceptable standards.

For each established indicator, criteria outline a quality-assessment strategy in terms of structure, process, and/or outcome measurement. The structured approach refers to the resource elements required to provide care. Since there is no strong correlation between structured criteria and the quality of care, professional energies should place particular emphasis on the development of process and outcome measures. Process criteria pertain to the activities of providing TR care while outcome criteria measure the consequences of TR intervention.

Developing Indicators and Criteria. The TR profession has established standards of practice that serve as a starting point for the design and implementation of quality-assessment activities in the field. However, they are generally limited to the structured approach and pertain little to elements of process and outcome. Because of this inherent weakness, standards should be used as a reference point to further develop indicators and criteria that are workable measures of the process and outcome of TR care.

Indicators are key areas or activities of a service requiring a specific quality-assessment focus. Depending on the specific characteristic of the TR program, many indicators might be identified as critical areas for quality monitoring and evaluation. Below is a sample list derived from the major aspects of TR care.

Indicators

Adequacy of Client Assessment	Client Goal Achievement
Quality of TR Intervention	Appropriate TR Intervention
Compliance w/ Policies & Standards	Completion of Program Plan
Quality of TR Treatment Plan	Adherence to Discharge Plan
Adequacy of Discharge Planning	Client Satisfaction
	Level of Participation

In a special article, Avedis Donabedian (1986) articulates guidelines useful in the development of criteria. (See Figure 6.4.) As TR criteria are re-

Figure 6.4 Guidelines for Criteria Development

Validity

Relevance to Outcome

Recordability

Acceptability to Case Variation

Stability and Timeliness

Stringency

Screening Efficiency

fined, special attention to validity and relevance issues are critical. The activities within the TR process must be coupled with expected outcomes so that these outcomes derive from TR intervention. Without this connection, claims upon the quality of care cannot be verified.

Criteria selection is contingent upon recording data from medical records on daily departmental reports. These data sources should be designed to efficiently access the quality-relevant information needed for criteria development. Additionally, the timing of data collection, depending on the patient risks involved, the frequency of service, and the volume of practice are important in determining when criteria can be employed.

Other factors include, first, the ability to change criteria over time as greater sophistication is obtained in professional practice. Second, the criteria should eschew the development of standards with unreasonable expectations but demand a level of quality consistent with professional consensus (stringency). Finally, criteria should tease out cases or service areas that require further screening.

Figure 6.5 shows an example indicator with respective criteria and standards for TR. For each criterion, the measurement strategy is specified, the acceptable standard defined, and the source of the data identified. Indicators may have more than one criteria statement, and the same criteria can be assigned to different indicators. Crucial in criteria development is the design of a valid measurement approach with related professional standards.

A Practitioner-based Approach. Academia has traditionally been charged with the responsibility of developing alternative approaches to TR. However, in the quality-assessment area, practitioners may be in the best position to conduct research and make inroads toward assessing quality. New strategies may be generated by practitioners on the line who are willing to "field test"

Figure 6.5 Criteria and Standards for Therapeutic Recreation

CRITERIA	STANDARD	MEASURE	DATA SOURCE
1. Clients whose discharge summary form is not completed with 24 hrs. of discharge.	5%	$\dfrac{\text{\# not done}}{\text{Total \# seen}}$	Record review
2. Clients with unresolved discharge problems.	10%	$\dfrac{\text{\# unresolved}}{\text{discharged}}$	Incident reports from utilization committee
3. Clients readmitted within 1 month of discharge.	10%	$\dfrac{\text{\# readmissions}}{\text{\# discharges}}$	Admission data
4. Clients dissatisfied with discharge process.	10%	$\dfrac{\text{\# dissatisfied}}{\text{\# discharges}}$	Client/family interview or survey

designs. Starting with the recreation body of knowledge and practice indicators, criteria and standards can be derived using the expertise and experience of in-house staff who are able to focus on the specific characteristics of their population, services, and delivery system. One method of developing indicators and criteria for your agency is to conduct a group exercise with your staff. Ask participants to draw on their own expertise to identify important aspects of TR care, formulate indicators, and specify the criteria and standards. Through a group-consensus process, quality-assessment monitoring activities can then be cultivated for your specific treatment setting.

For example, group members individually complete in stages the form in Figure 6.6 and then share their opinions with the group. First, staff list several major aspects of care and then collectively agree on one area to further pursue. Second, individuals develop indicators for the agreed-upon area, and, again as a group, identify one important quality-relevant indicator. Third, for each indicator, staff develop one criteria with related standards and measurement methods. Finally the group concurs on the most effective criteria, standards, and measures.

The methods stage requires determination of a sample size representative of the population yet realistic given available manpower resources. The group must also decide how frequently the indicator should be examined (see "timing" in Figure 6.4), how the data will be collected, what the data source is, and who will take responsibility for documenting and reporting the findings of the monitoring activity.

For this exercise to be successful, the group must come to a consensus at each stage before proceeding to the next level of discussion. The final outcome should be a quality-assessment activity representing the knowledge and experience of your staff that can be implemented as part of your QA pro-

Figure 6.6 Group Exercise Developing Quality Assessment Indicators and Criteria in Therapeutic Recreation

Major Aspects of Care: List 4 aspects of care in order of need for quality assessment (risk, frequency, and patient volume).

1. _____   2. _____

3. _____   4. _____

Indicator: Identify the indicator relating to the most important aspect of care.

Criteria: Develop objective, measurable criteria related to the indicator.

Standard: Specify states of criteria when acceptable quality is attained.

Methods: Sample size, frequency, staff responsibility and documentation.

Data Sources:

Adapted from *Quality Assurance in LTC*, (1986), JCAH.

gram. The exercise can be done numerous times, focusing on a different indicator of service and simultaneously distributing the role of facilitator among the staff. Figure 6.7 provides an example of the completed exercise.

Summary. The quality of a patient's care should be the singlemost important aspect of therapeutic recreation services. Through quality-assessment activities, the practitioner as well as the profession can address the "what," "how," and "when" of a comprehensive quality-assurance program. At the basic service level, professionals must be willing to take the initiative and examine the issues of indicator identification and appropriate measurement criteria. Such a grassroots approach is vitally important to the further development of

Figure 6.7 Group Exercise Developing Quality Assessment Indicators and Criteria in Therapeutic Recreation

Major Aspects of Care: List 4 aspects of care in order of need for quality assessment (risk, frequency, and patient volume).

1. _TR Intervention_   2. _____

3. _____   4. _____

Indicator: Identify the indicator relating to the most important aspect of care.

Client goal achievement

Criteria: Develop objective, measurable criteria related to the indicator.

Client whose goals are not achieved within original treatment plan.

Standard: Specify states of criteria when acceptable quality is attained.

20%   *# not achieved / total number*

Methods: Sample size, frequency, staff responsibility and documentation.

20% sample, monthly, supervisor or peer review team. QA summary form

Data Sources:

Patient records.

standards that are both outcome-based and appropriate for universal application in the field.

The viability of the TR profession is dependent on the quality of its services as perceived by both the provider and the client. Quality-assessment mechanisms which effectively monitor and evaluate the most important aspects of TR care must consider both these perspectives. Activities must also focus on efforts to measure both an acceptable level of patient satisfaction and the connection between the process and outcome of TR care.

Quality assurance is the conscience of the therapeutic-recreation profession. As the profession strives to improve the quality of TR services, it must be willing to move beyond the monitoring mechanisms that "assure" the quality of care and take aggressive steps toward "engineering" quality into all its services. The profession should be systematically planning for quality in TR practices by analyzing the dynamics of its practice patterns with respect to quality-of-care outcomes. Thus the development of indicators, criteria, and standards must proceed in unison with professional efforts to refine the techniques and methods of TR practice.

REFERENCES

Donabedian, A. (1986). "Criteria and Standards for Quality Assessment and Monitoring." *Quality Review Bulletin,* March.

Donabedian, A. (1982). *The Criteria and Standards of Quality.* Ann Arbor, MI: Health Administration Press.

Joint Commission on Accreditation of Hospitals (1986). *Quality Assurance in Long Term Care.* Chicago, IL.

VII. CLINICAL APPLICATION OF QUALITY ASSURANCE IN THE THERAPEUTIC RECREATION SETTING

ANN D. HUSTON

The evolution of quality assurance, within the past six years, has been dramatic and rapid with regard to the development of both standards and process. The 1979 state-of-the-art problem-focused evaluations are now simply considered the "problems of the month club." The major focus of quality assurance in 1986 is the monitoring and evaluation of clinical performance and quality of care. As therapeutic-recreation practitioners continue to address professional accountability issues, the maintenance of a sound quality-assurance program within individual service departments gains importance. This is due, in fact, to increased credibility and the provision of quality services. Professional accountability and the assurance of quality services must become synonymous to ensure that the highest level of therapeutic recreation services are provided. The existence of mandated standards by regulatory agencies as well as professional "competition" from other health-care disciplines should be recognized, yet should not be considered the sole reason for establishing a quality-assurance program.

A therapeutic-recreation department quality-assurance program must address a variety of clinical issues that are based upon the definition of "quality" provided by professional standards of practice and the interpretation of "assurance" provided by regulatory agencies. A quality-assurance program must be comprehensive in nature, addressing issues directly related to improving patient care and improving clinical performance. The most critical duty of the quality-assurance program is to cite opportunities that will improve patient care and the clinical performance of the therapeutic-recreation practitioner (JCAH, 1985). By prototype, a quality-assurance program is well planned, systematic, and ongoing as it monitors the routine, daily clinical functions of the practitioner and program. Therefore quality-assurance programs must be continually revised and evaluated at least annually. The inclusion of all clinical staff in the quality-assurance process is also encouraged to strengthen the validity of the entire quality-assurance process. Inviting clinical staff to assist in identifying existing or potential problems, detecting patterns or trends, and contributing to the resolution of such problems will assure their personal investment in quality and appropriateness of services. Resolution of identified problems, such as the implementation and follow-up of corrective action, is often overlooked. Nevertheless, it remains an important aspect of the quality-assurance process. If implementation of the corrective action does improve care or performance, as evidenced by the follow-up monitoring of the corrective action, then the quality-assurance process has been successful.

Institutional accreditation standards provide the basis for a continuous, systematic approach to the therapeutic-recreation quality-assurance program. However, such statements should not be regarded as all-inclusive. A variety of activities must be established within the therapeutic-recreation departmental quality-assurance program that address quality-care issues: utilization review; risk management; patient satisfaction; and annual department goals and objectives. The therapeutic-recreation quality-assurance program must be compatible with the institution's overall mission and objectives regarding quality assurance as well as remain consistent with professional standards of practice. Utilization of the written plan of operation, annual performance appraisals, position descriptions, and clinical privileges should also be included in the overall departmental quality-assurance program. (Examples of a recreation therapy quality assurance program are provided in Appendix A.)

Quality Assurance Program. When we address the Joint Commission on Accreditation of Hospitals (JCAH) quality-assurance standards, we see several critical elements repeatedly included in the five distinct accreditation programs. JCAH quality-assurance standards call for "on-going collection of data" (JCAH, 1985b) to support the monitoring and evaluation of the most important clinical functions. The on-going data-collection phase is one step identified as critical in the quality-assurance process because it assures quality and appropriateness of services. As previously mentioned, quality is defined utilizing key elements within the context of professional and medical-facility standards of practice. Appropriateness, likewise, is defined by the provision of therapeutic-recreation services based upon a multitude of variables relating to identified patient need and diagnosis.

With consideration to the overall quality-assurance program, regulatory standards, professional standards of practice, and "personality" of the medical facilities' provision of care, a framework for the quality-assurance plan may be developed to assist in the routine collection of data. A continuous and systematic quality-assurance program provides the structure necessary for daily monitoring and evaluation of the quality and appropriateness of therapeutic recreation services. Prior to the development of this "plan of action," the purpose of the therapeutic-recreation quality-assurance program must be identified. This statement of purpose should provide a concise, documented explanation of the functions of the department's quality-assurance program, including responsibilities and reporting mechanisms. (An example of a quality assurance mission statement for recreation therapy services is located in Appendix B.)

Quality Assurance Process. The success of a quality-assurance program is not simply the design of systematic, on-going collection of data, but the *process* involving continuous, systematic information-gathering. The development of monitoring and evaluating activities for the purpose of assuring quality and appropriateness of therapeutic-recreation services relies on five basic steps. These basic measures, if developed correctly, serve as the foundation for the monitoring activities of the annual quality-assurance program. First, identifying important aspects of care is essential in defining professional quality and appropriate services. Based upon these, more detailed indicators then must be identified to monitor quality and appropriateness— specifically the outcome of the important aspects of care. Objective criteria must then be established that further "indicate" expected outcomes. The collection of data, evaluation of this data, and communication of the findings combine for the fourth critical step in the process (JCAH, 1985b). The final step in monitoring and evaluating quality and appropriate services is the follow-up of the corrective action to assure improved patient care or clinical performance. The follow-up step is a return to the beginning of the monitoring process or the reinitiation of the entire cyclical process.

Identifying Elements of Care. Given the above stated outline (that quality is defined by key elements), the practitioner's initial step is identifying these key elements or important aspects of care. As previously mentioned, the involvement of clinical staff is extremely important in all stages of the quality-assurance process. Professional staff must collectively identify those aspects of care they consider most important. This should be done in relationship to the medical facility's mission statement and also consider the therapeutic-recreation services provided. Utilizing a variety of resources, such as professional standards of practice, accreditation standards, facility mission and policy statements, therapeutic-recreation philosophies, etc., the therapeutic-recreation practitioner will be able to identify the most important aspects of care provided. To compliment this identification process, the practitioner should ask several questions related to the provision of therapeutic recreation services:

1. What are the important functions of TR services?
2. What are necessary elements in the TR process?
3. What are my major responsibilities as a TR professional?
4. What indicates "quality" TR services to me?

Identification of the important clinical functions of a therapeutic-recreation program must be considered, such as assessment, program implementation, evaluation, patients' outcomes, etc. If the therapeutic-recreation practitioner can relate individual aspects of care to the issues of high risk or high volume, then it's possible that such aspects are good indicators of an important clinical function. For example, the completion of a clinical leisure assessment is a high-volume issue because the criteria specifies that leisure assessment will be completed on every new admission within seventy-two hours. An example of a high-risk issue would be the completion of an individual treatment plan based upon assessed need; the therapeutic-recreation practitioner is assuming risk for the independent development of an individual therapeutic-recreation treatment plan designed to meet specific leisure needs or dysfunctions. A final consideration in identifying important aspects of care are the issues of quality and appropriateness of therapeutic-recreation services. Questions the practitioner may ask that relate to issues of quality and appropriateness of care might include:

1. Will the collection of data provide information relative to quality services?
2. Does the information "indicate" the right service at the right time at the right intensity with the right person, etc.?

Practitioners must remember that identifying important aspects of care should not encompass specific therapeutic recreation procedures but rather generic aspects of quality and appropriate services. Generally, specifying three to six important aspects of care is sufficient to provide an adequate definition of quality therapeutic-recreation services. Examples of major clinical functions for therapeutic recreation services are provided in Appendix C.

Quality Assurance Plan. Planning individual quality-assurance activities is essential to assure systematic development and implementation of the overall quality-assurance program. Establishing an annual quality-assurance plan contributes to an organized, efficient and effective method of "assuring quality." Once you determine the clinically important aspects of care, you must plan individual activities that monitor and evaluate the care provided. These activities must specify: 1) the individual action to pursue; 2) the frequency of data collection and analysis of information; 3) the responsible staff person; and 4) whom the activity will involve (i.e., patient population), if appropriate. A well-planned, systematic, and comprehensive quality-assurance program is the cornerstone for the most efficient and effective approach to quality and appropriateness monitoring. The therapeutic-recreation practitioner will not suffer from extensive, prolonged quality-assurance "studies" or "audits" if he or she develops a well-planned system. (An example of an annual therapeutic recreation quality assurance plan is provided in Appendix D.)

Quality Indicators and Criteria. Upon identifying the important aspects of care and developing a systematic plan, you must establish specific indicators and criteria. These indicators are simply restated performance expectations and the desired outcome as a result of therapeutic intervention. Indicators represent the specific outcome resulting from quality and appropriate care. Similarly, development of specific criteria further details the expected performance or indicator. And clinically valid, objective criteria as a further delineation of expected performance and patient outcome are essential to the monitoring process. Utilizing both quality and appropriate indicators as well as objective criteria will assure quality clinical performances and appropriate therapeutic-recreation services.

Monitoring Process. Development of monitoring activities involves the important aspect of care, the indicators of quality and appropriateness, and the objective criteria that specify the minimum standard of expectation. (See Figure 7.1.) The planned routine collection of data must be supportive of the indicators and criteria established for each aspect of care. A proportionate number of monitoring activities (i.e., data collection and analysis) should be established for the selected indicators/criteria that are representative of quality and appropriate care. Analysis of the data must focus upon the improvement of clinical performance and patient care. Identification of isolated problems associated with care or performance is not the purpose of the routine quality-monitoring activity (JCAH, 1985). Problem-focused evaluations remain a function of the overall monitoring and evaluation process to assist with specific issues and problems. However, problem identification should not be the focal point of the quality-assurance program. (The monitoring and evaluation process is outlined in Appendix E.)

71

Figure 7.1 Monitoring and Evaluation

Monitoring Process

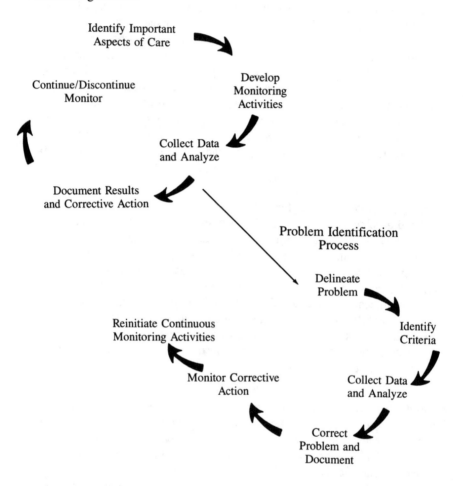

Documentation of the monitoring process, including the collection of data and analysis, is essential to determine the effectiveness of service as well as the establishment of trends or patterns of quality and appropriate care. Documentation can be used as an effective communication tool for many purposes within the quality-assurance process. Primarily, documentation is necessary to communicate the results internally through the facility's quality assurance chain of command, i.e., QA Coordinator, QA Committee, etc. Also, communicating results with the clinical staff in the therapeutic-recreation program is essential.

The importance of involving all clinical staff in the entire quality-assurance process cannot be overemphasized. Communication of data results and involvement of clinical staff in the interpretation of these results will strengthen the outcomes, the corrective action, and ultimately the clinical performance of the therapeutic-recreation practitioner. Upon identifying the necessity for corrective action, follow-up strategies should be established. Monitoring the corrective action, in essence, assures that such action was implemented and that patient care and clinical performance has improved as a direct result. Utilization of these results is often the "missing link" in the quality-assurance process. Assurance of quality and appropriateness of care cannot be determined without documented results of improvement. (For an example of the monitoring worksheet, refer to Appendix E.)

Problem Identification. As previously stated, the monitoring and evaluation process is the primary element in the quality-assurance plan. However, the problem-identification process also plays a significant role. (Refer to Figure 7.1.) The critical element of a sound quality-assurance program is the *process* that is maintained from beginning to end. The on-going collection of data should be constant. Through this continuous process the identification of specific problems requiring special attention is realized. Upon identifying a critical problem (from the continuous monitoring), you initiate a problem-focused evaluation that specifically addresses the cause of the significant problem. As in the monitoring and evaluation process, the identification of criteria, data collection and analysis, and implementation and evaluation of corrective action identifies both the problem and the necessary measures to correct the deficiency. Following success of the corrective action, the monitoring process is reinitiated.

Conclusion. Quality assurance is a highly individualized, independent, and critical function within therapeutic recreation. Routine quality-assurance activities that involve monitoring and evaluating the quality and appropriateness of care must be implemented to monitor program effectiveness, patient outcomes, and expected clinical performance. The therapeutic-recreation practitioner, while striving for professional credibility, must ask: 1) did the QA activity have an impact on patient care? 2) Did this process resolve a problem? If the answer to both these questions is "yes," then the quality-assurance activity has been successful in determining the quality and appropriateness of therapeutic-recreation services. (Appendix F provides four separate examples of monitoring activities that illustrate the QA process as presented in this paper.)

Monitoring activities demonstrate only one possible approach utilized at one specific medical facility. The reader is cautioned to investigate local standards of practice and the specific operation of the quality-assurance program within his or her medical facility. Therapeutic-recreation practitioners must independently identify quality-assurance programs, plans, activities, and reporting mechanisms relevant to their individual medical facility.

The implementation and maintenance of a sound quality-assurance program within therapeutic recreation will assist professionals as they strive for increased credibility within local medical facilities. Professional accountability within therapeutic recreation depends upon a number of variables, and the involvement of therapeutic-recreation practitioners in quality-assurance activities is an important step in achieving this goal. Therapeutic-recreation practitioners must not lose sight of the two critical elements in a quality-assurance activity: the improvement of clinical performance and the improvement of patient care. The ultimate goal of all quality-assurance programs must be to ensure the provision of the best possible therapeutic-recreation service. It is towards this end that we all must strive.

REFERENCES

Joint Commission on Accreditation of Hospitals (1985a). *An Introduction to JCAH: Its Survey, and Accreditation Process, Standards and Services.* Chicago, IL.

Joint Commission on Accreditation of Hospitals. (1985b). *Accreditation Manual for Hospitals.* Chicago, IL.

BIBLIOGRAPHY

Carruthers, C., Sneegas, J.F., & C. Ashton-Shaeffer, (1986). *Therapeutic Recreation Guidelines for Activity Services in Long Term Care.* Urbana-Champaign, IL: University of Illinois.

Coulton, C.F. (1986). "Implementing Monitoring and Evaluation Systems in Social Work." *Quality Review Bulletin, 2,* 72–75.

Craddick, J.W. (1983). *Medical Management Analysis: A Systematic Approach to Quality Assurance and Risk Management.*

Donabedian, A. (1986). "Criteria and Standards for Quality Assessment and Monitoring." *Quality Review Bulletin, 3,* 99–108.

Interqual (1984). *Clinical Support Services: Quality Monitoring and Appropriateness Evaluation,* 2nd Ed. North Hampton, NH.

Joint Commission on Accreditation of Hospitals (1985a). *An Introduction to JCAH: Its Survey, and Accreditation Process, Standards and Services.* Chicago, IL.

Joint Commission on Accreditation of Hospitals (1985b). *Accreditation Manual for Hospitals.* Chicago, IL.

Joint Commission on Accreditation of Hospitals (1985c). *Consolidated Standard Manual for Child, Adolescent, and Adult Psychiatric, Alcoholism, and Drug Abuse Facilities Serving the Mentally Retarded/Developmentally Disabled.* Chicago, IL.

Joint Commission on Accreditation of Hospitals (1985d). *Long Term Care Standards Manual.* Chicago, IL.

Joint Commission on Accreditation of Hospitals (1986a). *Quality Assurance in Long Term Care.* Chicago, IL.

Joint Commission on Accreditation of Hospitals (1986b). *JCAH Perspectives, 6,* 1–2.

National Therapeutic Recreation Society (1981). *Standards of Practice for Therapeutic Recreation Services.* Alexandria, VA: National Recreation and Park Association.

National Therapeutic Recreation Society (1982). *Philosophical Position Statement of the National Therapeutic Recreation Society.* Alexandria, VA: National Recreation and Park Association.

Navar, N., & J. Dunn, Eds. (1981). *Quality Assurance: Concerns for Therapeutic Recreation.* Urbana-Champaign, IL: University of Illinois.

Peterson, C.A. & S.L. Gunn, (1984). *Therapeutic Recreation, Program Design: Principles and Procedures*, 2nd Ed. Englewood Cliffs, NJ: Prentice-Hall, Inc.

Reynolds, R.P. & G. O'Morrow (1985). *Problems, Issues and Concepts in Therapeutic Recreation.* Englewood Cliffs, NJ: Prentice-Hall, Inc.

Veterans Administration Department of Medicine and Surgery (1986). Chief Medical Director Letter on Quality Assurance. Washington, DC.

APPENDIX A
RECREATION THERAPY
QUALITY ASSURANCE PROGRAM

Department Mission/Function Statement
Facility Mission/Function Statement
Organizational Charts
Activity Services Plan
Policy and Procedures
    Clinical Privileges
    Peer Review
    Clinical Staff Meetings
    Daily Recreation Activity Worksheets
    Infection Control
    Training and Development
    Medical Record Documentation
    Clinical Training and Affiliations
Monitoring and Evaluation Activities
Annual Goals and Objectives
Utilization Review
Minutes of Staff Meetings
Performance Standards
Position Descriptions
Patient Satisfaction Surveys
Management Briefings/Annual Reports

APPENDIX B
QUALITY ASSURANCE MISSION STATEMENT FOR RECREATION THERAPY SERVICES

The primary mission of the Recreation Therapy Service Quality Assurance Program is to assure the provision of efficient, effective, and qualitative therapeutic recreation services to the patient population based upon identified need. The objective is to maintain a systematic, continuous evaluation process that monitors the quality and appropriateness of therapeutic recreation services provided.

Quality therapeutic-recreation services are identified by the four major clinical activities or functions (attached) relative to the Veterans Administration and therapeutic recreation standards of practice. The evaluation process which is planned and ongoing includes criteria-based quality indicators that allow for clinically valid provision and utilization of therapeutic recreation services when indicated. Through the routine collection of data, the analysis, recommended action, and effectiveness of the action implemented, this process enables the recreation therapist to identify problem areas, need for improvement, and patterns or trends of the treatment services provided over time.

The entire recreation therapy staff is involved in the planning, implementation, and evaluation of this quality-assurance program at varying participative levels based upon the individual's demonstrated clinical competence. The Service Chief assumes administrative responsibility for the assignment and completion of the quality-assurance activities—routine or exceptional.

The methodology of this process involves the routine collection of information by a responsible staff person to develop a sufficient data base that allows for objective clinical analysis in determining the quality and appropriateness of therapeutic recreation services. Following assessment of the data collected, necessary measures will be identified and implemented to correct and/or improve clinical performance. An essential, final component will be the evaluation and documentation of action items implemented, the effectiveness and impact on patient treatment as a result of each action item.

APPENDIX C
MAJOR CLINICAL FUNCTIONS FOR THERAPEUTIC RECREATION SERVICE

ASSESSMENT AND CLINICAL ANALYSIS OF LEISURE DYSFUNCTION

TREATMENT MODALITIES AND INTERVENTIONS BASED UPON ASSESSED
        LEISURE FUNCTIONAL NEEDS
        LEISURE EDUCATIONAL NEEDS
        SELF-DIRECTED LEISURE NEEDS

TREATMENT EVALUATION AND DISCHARGE PLANNING

PROFESSIONAL DEVELOPMENT AND TRAINING

APPENDIX D
ANNUAL THERAPEUTIC
RECREATION QUALITY
ASSURANCE PLAN

RECREATION THERAPY SERVICE QUALITY ASSURANCE PLAN—1986
V.A. MEDICAL CENTER, KANSAS, MISSOURI

ASSESSMENT AND CLINICAL ANALYSIS OF LEISURE DYSFUNCTION

	Jan	Feb	Mar	Apr	May	Jun	Jul	Aug	Sep	Oct	Nov	Dec	Staff Responsible	Remarks
Timeliness of assessments	+	+	*	+	+	*	+	+	*	+	+	*	Svc. Chief	
Appropriateness of treatment flow	*							*					Svc. Chief	
Appropriateness of clinical summary indicators			+				+				+		Svc. Chief	
Timeliness of responses upon admission								*				*	Svc. Chief	
Appropriateness of assessment entries								+	+	*			Svc. Chief	
Appropriateness of ADTU activity evaluations	+			@	+		@	+	+		@		Svc. Chief	
R T involvement in master treatment plan			*			*			*			*	Svc. Chief	

KEY:
+ — data collection
@ — data analysis
* — collection and analysis

TREATMENT MODALITIES AND INTERVENTIONS BASED UPON
ASSESSED: LEISURE FUNCTIONAL NEEDS
LEISURE EDUCATION NEEDS
SELF-DIRECTED LEISURE NEEDS

	Jan	Feb	Mar	Apr	May	Jun	Jul	Aug	Sep	Oct	Nov	Dec	Staff Responsible	Remarks
R.T. involvement in treatment plan reviews		*			*			*				*	Staff	Assignments on Rotating Basis
Program Review and Evaluation														
—Peer review of program objectives					+			*			+		Staff	
—Interventions and objectives coincide				*						*			Staff	
PTU's by discipline and modality			*			*			*			*	Svc. Chief	
Appropriateness of self-directed leisure programs			+		+		+	@					Staff	Monitor 1st week—1st month,
Activities resulting in the filing of incident reports	+	+	@										Staff	2nd week—2nd month, and 3rd week—3rd month

RECREATION THERAPY SERVICE QUALITY ASSURANCE PLAN
1986
V.A. MEDICAL CENTER, KANSAS, MISSOURI

TREATMENT EVALUATION AND DISCHARGE PLANNING

	Jan	Feb	Mar	Apr	May	Jun	Jul	Aug	Sep	Oct	Nov	Dec	Staff Responsible	Remarks
Timeliness of discharge plans	+	+	*	+	+	*	+	+	*	+	+	*	Svc. Chief	
R.T. involvement in team discharge plans			+	@					+		*		Svc. Chief	
Discharge recommendation components			+		+		+		+		+		Staff	
Discharge plans coincide with TR indications		+	@										Staff	
Discontinuance of treatment prior to discharge			+	@						+	@		Staff	

PROFESSIONAL DEVELOPMENT AND TRAINING

	Jan	Feb	Mar	Apr	May	Jun	Jul	Aug	Sep	Oct	Nov	Dec	Staff Responsible	Remarks
Educational needs assessment									+	@			Svc. Chief	(and staff)
Past training needs evaluation											*		Svc. Chief	
Review of clinical performance				*							*	*	Svc. Chief	
(via professional standards)													Staff	
Peer review of clinical treatment components														
a. assessments									*			*	Staff	
b. treatment plans						*							Staff	
c. discharge plans													Staff	
d. treatment flow			*										Staff	
Student program compliance evaluation										+	+	*	Intern Supervisor	(when established)

APPENDIX E
MONITORING AND EVALUATION PROCESS

RECREATION THERAPY SERVICE QUALITY ASSURANCE PLAN MONITOR
WORKSHEET

PART I

MAJOR CLINICAL FUNCTION

PURPOSE OF MONITOR

SAMPLE

METHODOLOGY

COMPLIANCE INDICATORS

OBJECTIVE CRITERIA

PART II

SUMMARY OF MONITOR

ANALYSIS OF FINDINGS

RECOMMENDATIONS

ACTION STEPS

APPENDIX F
RECREATION THERAPY
MONITORING ACTIVITY
WORKSHEETS

WORKSHEET 1

MAJOR CLINICAL FUNCTION: Treatment Modalities and Interventions Based Upon:
    Leisure Functional Needs,
    Leisure Educational Needs,
    Self-directed Leisure Needs

PURPOSE OF MONITOR: To determine the recreation therapists' involvement in the multidisciplinary treatment plan reviews as well as to assure recreation-therapy plan input and documentation in these reviews.

SAMPLE: Five records from each treatment team

METHODOLOGY: Chief, Recreation Therapy Service, will review the medical-record master-treatment plan reviews completed on each patient monthly.

COMPLIANCE INDICATORS: Eighty percent involvement by each recreation therapist is minimum level of compliance during scheduled monitoring activity.

OBJECTIVE CRITERIA: Criteria established in Recreation Therapy Service Policy and Procedure Manual/Intra Office Memorandum No. 12. Additionally, the recreation therapist will establish a mechanism to assure inclusion of the recreation therapy treatment plan in every master treatment plan review. Mandatory attendance in one multidisciplinary treatment team meeting each week.

1. Recreation therapy treatment plan/activities will be listed in the MTP review (either by the recreation therapist or the treatment team leader).

2. The recreation therapists' attendance at the meetings is documented along with other treatment-team members per Medical Center Memorandum 11-85-38.

3. The recreation therapist will sign each review verifying concurrence with MTP review as established by the multidisciplinary treatment team.

SUMMARY OF MONITOR: Data reviewed included the recreation therapist's involvement in the Master Treatment Plan Reviews completed by unit multidisciplinary treatment teams. Randomly reviewed twenty percent of ADC on 10 East, 10 West, and Day Hospital during this month, with eighty percent involvement of recreation therapist compliance.

ANALYSIS OF FINDINGS: Only one treatment plan review did not include mention of the recreation therapy activities or indicate the recreation therapist's involvement in the planning process. All other review plans indicated compliance with identifying primary treatment problems related to leisure, the recreation therapist's participation in the treatment, planning, and signature.

ACTION: No action necessary.

FOLLOW-UP: None.

Data Collection

R.T. INVOLVEMENT IN MTP REVIEWS

CRITERIA #1   R.T. plan/activities are listed in MTP review (by R.T. or Leader)

CRITERIA #2   R.T. attendance at MDT meetings

CRITERIA #3   R.T. signature

Patient name	SS#	Unit	CRITERIA 1	2	3	COMMENTS

WORKSHEET 2

MAJOR CLINICAL FUNCTION: Professional Development and Training

PURPOSE OF MONITOR: To collect data regarding peer review of individual treatment components, specifically the comprehensive leisure-assessment components and the appropriateness of the entries in the medical record.

SAMPLE: Twenty percent average daily census during September (N = 12)

METHODOLOGY: Recreation therapists assigned to September rotation to Service Peer Review Program complete peer review as designed in Recreation Therapy Service Policy and Procedure Manual/Intra Office Memorandum No. 13.

COMPLIANCE INDICATORS: Ninety percent acceptable compliance

OBJECTIVE CRITERIA: Criteria as established in Intra Office Memorandum No. 13 "Peer Review Program" (see attached).

Recreation Therapy Service Peer/Supervisory Review Form

Patient Name: SS#:

Reviewers: Unit:

Date: Rating Comments & Qualifiers

Compliance Key:

1. Assessment

    a. Past leisure interest

        1. Past leisure pursuits

        2. Frequency of involvement or

        *3. Qualifiers for lack of information

    b. Current leisure interest

        1. Current leisure interest

        2. Frequency of participation (weekly, monthly)

        3. Leisure time usage prior to admission (up to 1 year)

        *4. Use of leisure time on ward

    c. Socialization Level

        1. Ability to initiate conversation

        2. Ability to maintain eye contact

    *3. Ability to function in small or large groups

    *4. Ability to seek out others in leisure

    5. Barrier to leisure dysfunction or asset qualified
by highest level of function

d. Attention Span

    1. Orientation to time, place, person

    2. Ability to stay on tasks

    *3. Response to interviewer (i.e., quick or delayed, rational or irrational)

    4. Barrier to leisure dysfunction or asset qualified
by highest level of functioning

e. Physical Disabilities

    1. Require adaptation to leisure or

    2. Require attention during treatment

    *3. Activity/inactivity level

    *4. Medical information from chart

    5. Barrier to leisure dysfunction or asset qualified
by highest level of functioning

f. Funding Level

    1. Extent of finances for leisure

    2. Attitude of patient using personal funds for leisure

    *3. Extent of limitation/adaptation for leisure

    4. Barrier to leisure dysfunction for asset qualified
by highest level of functioning

    *5. Transportation availability/awareness (statement)

g. Motivation Level

    1. Willingness to participate in treatment recommendations

    2. Level of recognition of person and leisure needs

    3. Level of leisure understanding (i.e., leisure definition, examples)

    4. Attitude towards positive leisure lifestyle

    *5. Extrinsic motivation

    6. Barrier to leisure dysfunction or asset qualified
by highest level of functioning

h. Clinical Impression

   1. Summary of clinical findings

   2. Prioritized leisure barriers and strengths

   3. Level of leisure functioning

   4. Discharge prognosis

   5. Discharge recommendations/plan

i. Short Range Goals

   1. Written in measurable/behavioral terms

   2. Task specific

   3. Intensity/frequency of interventions

   4. Treatment time frame

   5. Reflects primary leisure barrier

j. Long Range Goals

   1. Generalization of desired treatment outcomes

   2. Reflects the established discharge plan

k. Treatment Plan

   1. Specific treatment modalities

   2. Frequency of treatment interventions

   3. Relationship to goal

EVALUATION OF OVERALL CONTENT

Needs Improvement	Satisfactory	Above Average	Outstanding
(1 – 6)	(6 – 11)	(11 – 17)	(17 – 22)

COMMENTS: (Use back if necessary)

0–4 Missed the Boat
5–6 Average
7–8 Above Average

l. Interim Note   Rating Comments & Qualifers

   1. Diagnosis stated

   2. Note within 3 weeks

   3. Written in SOAP format

   4. Short-range goal stated

5. Interventions or modalities stated

6. Progress note towards goal

7. New goal stated

8. Plan started if amended

II. Final Note

1. Diagnosis stated

2. Written in 2 days after discharge

3. Current goal stated

4. Summary of treatment:

   a. Interventions or modalities used.

   b. Patient's response to treatment.

5. Patient's discharge plan

6. Therapist's recommendations

III. COMMENTS: (of overall continuity of treatment from assessment to discharge plan)

SUMMARY OF MONITOR: Peer review of clinical-treatment components that specifically indicate appropriate comprehensive leisure assessments and utilize the peer-review-criteria worksheet. Six records were reviewed with established compliance as ninety percent assessment categories completed appropriately.

ANALYSIS OF FINDINGS: All assessment categories completed as indicated, however, specific indicators within generic categories were consistently excluded due to the establishment of new quality indicators in the assessment procedure this month.

ACTION: Review during second quarter FY 86 following adequate time to implement newly established quality indicators.

FOLLOW-UP: February 1986

WORKSHEET 3

MAJOR CLINICAL FUNCTION: Treatment Evaluation and Discharge Planning

PURPOSE OF MONITOR: To determine if the timeliness of discharge plans are consistent with established standards, thus to ensure appropriate recreation-therapy input into the discharge process.

SAMPLE: One hundred percent of patients discharged during the month August from 10 East, 10 West, and Day Hospital

METHODOLOGY: Chief, Recreation Therapy Service, will review all discharge plans to determine timeliness of entry into medical record.

COMPLIANCE INDICATORS: Ninety percent of all discharge plans completed in a timely manner as the Service goal.

OBJECTIVE CRITERIA: Criteria established in Recreation Therapy Service Policy and Procedure Manual/Intra Office Memorandum No. 12 "Medical Record Documentation." (Time requirements state that the discharge final plan will be entered into the medical record prior to the patient's discharge but no later than two days following the discharge.)

1. Discharge Date

2. Date of Discharge Plan

3. Days Elapsed (see attached)

Data Collection

TIMELINESS OF DISCHARGE PLANS

CRITERIA #1   Date of Discharge

CRITERIA #2   Date of Discharge Plan

CRITERIA #3   Days Elapsed

DISCHARGES

	Before Discharge	on D/C	1–3 days after	4–5 days	+++
REC. THERAPIST 1 81% = 32/41					
REC THERAPIST 2 70% = 9/13					
REC THERAPIST 3 100% = 40/40					

Service Percentage: 59/70 = 86%

SUMMARY OF MONITOR: Timeliness of discharge plans for one hundred percent of patients discharged from 10 East, 10 West, and Day Hospital. Service policy indicates discharge plans will be entered into the medical record no later than two days following discharge. Service goal is ninety percent.

ANALYSIS OF FINDINGS:

Therapist 1 — 32/41 = 81% compliance
Therapist 2 — 9/13 = 70% compliance
Therapist 3 — 40/40 = 100% compliance

ACTION: Continue monitor according to Service plan.

FOLLOW-UP: March 1986 — Service Chief.

WORKSHEET 4

MAJOR CLINICAL FUNCTION: Assessment and Clinical Analysis of Leisure Dysfunction

PURPOSE OF MONITOR: To determine the appropriateness of the treatment flow as documented in the patient's medical record. To assure treatment programs are established according to patient's leisure needs, barriers, capacities, etc., as assessed.

SAMPLE: All patients assessed on 10 East, 10 West, and Day Hospital for two weeks (fourteen working days), August 11-25, 1985.

METHODOLOGY: All assessments during time frames will be reviewed by the Chief, Recreation Therapy Service. The clinical summaries, treatment goals, and objectives, as well as the treatment plans, will be examined for inter-relationships and consistency of treatment planned.

COMPLIANCE INDICATORS: Ninety to ninety-five percent compliance on all assessments reviewed.

OBJECTIVE CRITERIA

	REHAB.	LEIS. ED.	VOLUN.
1. Clinical impression identifies pts. functional level with prioritization of dysfunctions.			
2. Treatment goals coincide w/ functional level (addressing specific dysfunction identified).			
3. Treatment plan defines a specific treatment regime to meet identified functional level (and specific dysfunction).			

SUMMARY REPORT

Report of:

Department/Service: Recreation Therapy

Reporting Time Frame: (Check One)   —— Annually   —— Semiannually
                                      —— Quarterly —— Monthly

DATA EXAMINED	ASSESSMENT FINDINGS	ACTION	FOLLOW-UP WHAT/WHEN/RESULTS
1. Timeliness of Comprehensive Leisure Assessments	Therapist I — (12/38) 32% compliance Therapist II — (15–17) 88% compliance Therapist III — (36/36) 100% compliance Service — 69% compliance (goal is 85%)	1. Initiate problems-focused evaluation on Therapist I. Continue to monitor.	
2. Timeliness of Discharge Plans	Therapist I — (23/31) 68% compliance Therapist II — (7/10) 70% compliance Therapist III — (29/29) 100% compliance Service (59/70) 84% compliance (goal is 90%)	Continue to monitor.	

SUMMARY REPORT (CONT'D)

DATA EXAMINED	ASSESSMENT FINDINGS	ACTION	FOLLOW-UP WHAT/WHEN/RESULTS
3. ADTU Activity Evaluations	January review — a. 11 records reviewed: 9 of 11 contained completed evaluations. 2 of 11 patients AMA D/C prior to 10-day deadline 6 of 11 records completed within 10 days of admission. 82% compliance.	Forward to ADTU Coordinator for follow-up.	

VIII. QUALITY ASSURANCE FOR THERAPEUTIC RECREATION: CLOSING REMARKS

RAY WEST

After participating in the presentations over the past several days, the impression I am left with is one of quality. The seminar was extremely well-organized and the information presented was progressive. I am impressed by the depth of the information on quality assurance and the fact that much of it is current and state-of-the-art. I am also pleased with the level of involvement of the participants. Your diligence and commitment to discussing a complex issue in an in-depth way over the past several days has been outstanding. In addition, I am excited about what I think are the beginnings of a new emphasis on quality assurance for therapeutic recreation.

In my opening remarks, I talked about the evolution of the therapeutic-recreation profession and the many professional issues we face. I also spoke about the evolution of health care and, in particular, the rate of change in the health-care industry. This rate exceeds that of our profession; therefore therapeutic recreation is not keeping pace and may be falling behind. To keep this from happening, I identified several key points which I hoped would guide some of our discussions about quality assurance relative to therapeutic recreation, including the following:

- We must demonstrate the efficacy of our service to survive.
- We must measure the outcome of our service for our clients and for the service system of which we are a part.

- We must make quality assurance a primary and major focus of our profession.

Effective quality assurance is probably the best way to address our many professionalization efforts, and it can be the foundation for several activities, including:

1. Further discussion of philosophy and definitions,
2. Expansion of our literature and body of knowledge,
3. Development and compliance with standards,
4. Certification, as well as many other professionalization issues.

In short, quality assurance should be the foundation upon which we build a service profession.

In several recent presentations, I have made reference to a publication entitled *In Search of Excellence* (1982). I think it should be of interest to our profession since it identifies many commonly shared characteristics and principles that have enabled outstanding companies or businesses to survive and be successful over the long run. If in our professionalization efforts we are to turn our thinking from the short-term to the long-term, many of these principles can have applications for us. Two in particular might benefit therapeutic recreation. The first, "staying close to the customer," means that excellent companies know what they perceive about their products and services and what they want to have delivered in terms of products and services. Relative to therapeutic recreation, we have several customers or consumers, including patients and clients, physicians, administrators, third-party payers, allied health disciplines, etc. It is very important that we stay close to our customers/consumers and understand what they perceive us to be and desire us to be, and what services they want us to deliver. A second principle is that excellent companies are "hands on, value driven." This means that successful businesses are driven by values shared at all levels of the organization from the bottom to the top. These values are understood, accepted, shared, and espoused by those in direct-service delivery, and have obvious application for the quality of the products or services delivered.

On the drive here from the airport, Rich Hoffman and I had a discussion about our profession and the health-care industry. We determined that we are "professionals" or "technicians" depending on how we deliver services. According to Carol Peterson (1981), a professional has some distinguishing attributes and characteristics:

> A professional has an established and recognized set of skills and a body of knowledge that is implemented in a consistent manner, resulting in the delivery of services that are recognized for their quality and predictable impact; in addition, the professional is a

part of a collective group of others who regulate themselves and the services they provide as a whole, so that the consumer can expect and rely upon their judgment, motivations, procedures, and product.

I think this statement has many implications for our growing involvement in quality assurance and our collective activities as a profession. If we are professionals, clients and consumers will be able to depend on the quality and predictable impact of the services that we deliver. If we are professionals, we will be a part of a collective group who regulate ourselves to ensure the quality of services provided.

At the beginning of this conference I challenged the group to be aggressive in pursuing quality assurance. That challenge is still before us. We must continue, not only this morning, but when we leave here, to actively pursue the issue of quality assurance. If we lose sight of the necessity to deliver quality service to our clients, we are lost. On the job we won't be able to accomplish quality assurance in a day, a week, or possibly even a month. It has to be a primary focus of *all* we do. In our profession, it will also take time for us to collectively work together on the issue of quality assurance. The challenge remains . . . let's work together as a profession to ensure quality of service for our consumers.

REFERENCES

Peters, J. and Waterman, R. (1982). *In Search of Excellence*. New York, NY: Warner Books, Inc.

Peterson, C.A. (1981). "Pride and Progress Professionalization." In G. Hitzhusen (Ed.). *Expanding Horizons in Therapeutic Recreation VII*. Columbia, MO: University of Missouri, pp. 1–9.

IX. EPILOGUE: FUTURE PERSPECTIVE ON THERAPEUTIC RECREATION QUALITY ASSURANCE

This book is designed to provide the reader with an understanding of the concepts and application of quality assurance as it pertains to the therapeutic recreation process. Each author, in presenting his or her view, also presented, implicitly or explicitly, a unique perception of the meaning and definition of the QA process. Total consensus as to what constitutes QA is rare among health care professionals. This is quite evident among therapeutic recreation professionals as well.

Amid the confusion that surrounds the QA debate is one generally accepted fact: QA, and the emphasis placed upon it by regulatory agencies, will continue to dominate the health care arena for decades to come. As such, accountability, cost containment and risk management will persist as key obstacles to the growth of therapeutic recreation. Acceptance of therapeutic recreation professionalism by the general health care community depends squarely on the ability of therapeutic recreation to demonstrate effective and efficient service. It is toward this end that future QA efforts need to aim.

Although this publication represents an encouraging beginning, the road ahead is long and steep. Efforts to monitor and evaluate the progress of quality assurance in therapeutic recreation must continue. National forums, such as the one that served as the impetus for this book, should be sponsored on both a timely and regular basis. Research projects, encouraged and supported by national professional associations, should commence in a strategic effort to keep pace with allied health-profession groups.

Paramount among short-range objectives for QA in therapeutic recreation is the development and adoption of outcome-based measurement approaches. Most recently, the Joint Commission of Accreditation of Hospitals and the American Medical Association have called for widespread adoption of such measures. Due in part to the lack of supportive efficacy studies, they perceive the use of such assessment strategies in therapeutic recreation as most challenging.

On the management front, the integration of QA into the therapeutic recreation system is also paramount. Outcome data must be incorporated into other areas of evaluation, including productivity analysis and personnel evaluation. Quality Assurance mechanisms should also help determine professional privileging.

In the area of professional preparation and professional competency, individuals who are awarded degrees and certification in therapeutic recreation should be competent in the quality assurance process. This may mean that potential professionals receive more concentrated coursework in evaluation methodology and statistical analysis.

Lastly, concentrated efforts are necessary to develop and validate a model QA program for therapeutic recreation. Such a model should address the essential elements of therapeutic recreation service, and serve as a link between certification and standards of practice. The linkage established among these three essential components of professionalism would tremendously enhance therapeutic recreation's position within the health care environment.

The future of quality assurance is uncertain with respect to direction, but not so with respect to importance. Increasingly, therapeutic recreation professionals will be called upon to report their own quality assessment activities, and to justify their role within the health care environment. To a large degree the success of such actions will be determined by our collective individual actions in addressing the QA issue today. By following the strategies outlined above, we should realize the ultimate goal of providing top-notch therapeutic recreation services.

I hope the outcomes of our efforts are of a high quality.

BOB RILEY

OTHER BOOKS FROM VENTURE PUBLISHING

Leisure In Your Life: An Exploration, Revised Edition, by Geoffrey Godbey

Recreation and Leisure: Issues In An Era of Change, Revised Edition, edited by Thomas L. Goodale and Peter A. Witt

Recreation Economic Decisions: Comparing Benefits and Costs, by Richard G. Walsh

Acquiring Parks and Recreation Facilities Through Mandatory Dedication: A Comprehensive Guide, by Ronald A. Kaiser and James D. Mertes

Planning Parks for People, by John Hultsman, Richard L. Cottrell and Wendy Zales Hultsman

Private and Commercial Recreation, edited by Arlin Epperson

Sports and Recreation: An Economic Analysis, by Chris Gratton and Peter Taylor (Distributed for E. and F.N. Spon, Ltd., London, England)

Park Ranger Handbook, by J.W. Shiner

Leadership and Administration of Outdoor Pursuits, by Phyllis Ford and James Blanchard

Marketing Parks and Recreation, by National Park Service

Vandalism Control Management for Parks and Recreation Areas, by Monty L. Christiansen

Playing, Living, Learning — A Worldwide Perspective on Children's Opportunities to Play, by Cor Westland and Jane Knight

International Directory of Academic Institutions in Recreation Leisure and Related Fields (Distributed for WLRA)